UNDERGROUND
CLINICAL VIGNETTES

PEDIATRICS

D0483348

Classic Clinical Cases for
USMLE Step 2 Review [56 cases]

VIKAS BHUSHAN, MD
University of California, San Francisco, Class of 1991
Series Editor, Diagnostic Radiologist

TAO LE, MD
University of California, San Francisco, Class of 1996
Yale-New Haven Hospital, Resident in Internal Medicine

CHIRAG AMIN, MD
University of Miami, Class of 1996
Orlando Regional Medical Center, Resident in Orthopaedic Surgery

JOSE M. FIERRO, MD
Brookdale Hospital, Resident in Medicine/Pediatrics

HOANG NGUYEN
Northwestern University, Class of 2000

VISHAL PALL, MBBS
Government Medical College, Chandigarh, India, Class of 1996

NOTICE

The authors of this volume have taken care that the information contained herein is accurate and compatible with the standards generally accepted at the time of publication. Nevertheless, it is difficult to ensure that all the information given is entirely accurate for all circumstances. The publisher and authors do not guarantee the contents of this book and disclaim liability, loss, or damage incurred as a consequence, directly or indirectly, of the use and application of any of the contents of this volume.

DISTRIBUTED by Blackwell Science, Inc.
Editorial Office:
Commerce Place, 350 Main Street, Malden, Massachusetts 02148, USA

DISTRIBUTORS

USA

Commerce Place
350 Main Street
Malden, Massachusetts 02148
(Telephone orders: 800-215-1000 or
781-388-8250;
fax orders: 781-388-8270)

Canada

Login Brothers Book Company
324 Saulteaux Crescent
Winnipeg, Manitoba, R3J 3T2
(Telephone orders: 204-224-4068;
Telephone: 800-665-1148;
fax: 800-665-0103

Australia

Blackwell Science Pty Ltd.
54 University Street
Carlton, Victoria 3053
(Telephone orders: 03-9347-0300;
fax orders: 03-9349-3016)

Outside North America and Australia

Blackwell Science, Ltd.
c/o Marston Book Service, Ltd.
P.O. Box 269
Abingdon
Oxon OX14 4YN
England
(Telephone orders: 44-01235-465500;
fax orders: 44-01235-465555)

ISBN: 1-890061-21-2
TITLE: Underground Clinical Vignettes: Pediatrics

Editor: Andrea Fellows
Typesetter: Vikas Bhushan using MS Word97
Printed and bound by Capital City Press

Printed in the United States of America
99 00 01 02 6 5 4 3 2 1

Contributors

NAVNEET DHILLON, MBBS
Government Medical College, Chandigarh, Class of 1997

LINH NGUYEN, MD
University of Illinois, Chicago, Resident in Surgery

VIPAL SONI
UCLA School of Medicine, Class of 1999

ASHRAF ZAMAN, MBBS
International Medical Graduate

Faculty Reviewer

THAO PHAM, MD
Yale-New Haven Hospital, Resident in Pediatrics

Acknowledgments

. . . .

Throughout the production of this book, we have had the support of many friends and colleagues. Special thanks to our business manager, Gianni Le Nguyen. For expert computer support, Tarun Mathur and Alex Grimm. For additional copy editing services, Erica Simmons. For design suggestions, Sonia Santos and Elizabeth Sanders.

For authorship, editing, proofreading, and assistance across the vignette series, we collectively thank Chris Aiken, Kris Alden, Ted Amanios, Henry Aryan, Natalie Barteneva, MD, Adam Bennett, Ross Berkeley, MD, Archana Bindra, MBBS, Sanjay Bindra, MBBS, Aminah Bliss, Tamara Callahan, MD, MPP, Aaron Caughey, MD, MPP, Deanna Chin, Vladimir Coric, MD, Vladimir Coric, Sr., MD, Ronald Cowan, MD, PhD, Ryan Crowley, Daniel Cruz, Zubin Damania, Rama Dandamudi, MD, Sunit Das, Brian Doran, MD, Alea Eusebio, Thomas Farquhar, Jose Fierro, MBBS, Tony George, MD, Parul Goyal, Sundar Jayaraman, Eve Kaiyala, Sudhir Kakarla, Seth Karp, MD, Bertram Katzung, MD, PhD, Aaron Kesselheim, Jeff Knake, Sharon Kreijci, Christopher Kosgrove, MD, Warren Levinson, MD, PhD, Eric Ley, Joseph Lim, Andy Lin, Daniel Lee, Scott Lee, Samir Mehta, Gil Melmed, Michael Murphy, MD, MPH, Dan Neagu, MD, Deanna Nobleza, Craig Nodurft, Henry Nguyen, Linh Nguyen, MD, Vishal Pall, MBBS, Paul Pamphrus, MD, Thao Pham, MD, Michelle Pinto, Riva Rahl, Aashita Randeria, Rachan Reddy, Rajiv Roy, Diego Ruiz, Sanjay Sahgal, MD, Mustafa Saifee, MD, Louis Sanfillipo, MD, John Schilling, Sonal Shah, Nutan Sharma, MD, PhD, Andrew Shpall, Kristy Smith, Tanya Smith, Vipal Soni, Brad Spellberg, Merita Tan, MD, Eric Taylor, Jennifer Ty, Anne Vu, MD, Eunice Wang, MD, Lynna Wang, Andy Weiss, Thomas Yoo, and Ashraf Zaman, MBBS. Please let us know if your name has been missed or misspelled and we will be happy to make the change in the next edition.

For generously contributing images to the entire *Underground Clinical Vignette* Step 2 series, we collectively thank the staff at Blackwell Science in Oxford, Boston, and Berlin as well as:

- Alfred Cuschieri, Thomas P.J. Hennessy, Roger M. Greenhalgh, David I. Rowley, Pierce A. Grace (*Clinical Surgery*, © 1996 Blackwell Science), Figures 13.23, 13.35b, 13.51, 15.13, 15.2.

- John Axford (*Medicine*, © 1996 Blackwell Science), Figures f 3.10, 2.103a, 2.110b, 3.20a, 3.20b, 3.25b, 3.38a, 5.9Bi, 5.9Bii, 6.41a, 6.41b, 6.74b, 6.74c, 7.78ai, 7.78aii, 7.78b, 8.47b, 9.9e, f 3.17, f 3.36, f 3.37, f 5.27, f 5.28, f 5.45a, f 5.48, f 5.49a, f 5.50, f 5.65a, f 5.67, f 5.68, f 8.27a, AX10.120b, 11.63b, 11.63c, 11.68a, 11.68b, 11.68c, 12.37a, 12.37b.

Table of Contents

. . . .

Preface

. . . .

This series was developed to address the nearly universal presence of clinical vignette questions on the USMLE Step 2. It is designed to supplement and complement *First Aid for the USMLE Step 2* (Appleton & Lange). Bidirectional cross-linking to appropriate High-Yield Facts in the second edition of *First Aid for the USMLE Step 2* has been implemented.

Each book uses a series of approximately 50 **"supra-prototypical" cases as a way to condense testable facts and associations.** The clinical vignettes in this series are designed to incorporate as many testable facts as possible into a cohesive and memorable clinical picture. The vignettes represent composites drawn from general and specialty textbooks, reference books, thousands of USMLE-style questions and the personal experience of the authors and reviewers. Additionally, we present "Associated Diseases" as a way to teach the most critical facts about a larger number of diseases that do not justify an entire case. **The "Associated Diseases" list is NOT complete and does not represent differential diagnoses.**

Although each case tends to present all the signs, symptoms, and diagnostic findings for a particular illness, **patients generally will not present with such a "complete" picture either clinically or on the Step 2 exam.** Cases are not meant to simulate a potential real patient or an exam vignette. All the **boldfaced "buzzwords" are for learning purposes** and are not necessarily expected to be found in any one patient with the disease. **Similarly, the images for each case are for learning purposes only, were derived from a variety of textbooks, and may not match the clinical vignette in all respects.** Images are labeled [A]–[D] and represent 1–4 images of varying sizes, with locations corresponding to a left-to-right, top-to-bottom lettering system.

Definitions of selected important terms are placed within the vignettes in (= SMALL CAPS) in parentheses. Other parenthetical remarks often refer to the pathophysiology or mechanism of disease. The format should also help students learn to present cases succinctly during oral "bullet" presentations on clinical rotations. The cases are meant to be read as a condensed review, not as a primary reference.

The information provided in this book has been prepared with a great deal of thought and careful research. This book should not, however, be considered your sole source of information. Corrections, suggestions, and submissions of new cases are encouraged and will be acknowledged and incorporated in future editions.

Abbreviations

. . . .

ABGs - arterial blood gases
ACTH - adrenocorticotropic hormone
ADA - adenosine deaminase
AIDS - acquired immunodeficiency syndrome
ALL - acute lymphocytic leukemia
ALT - alanine transaminase
AMP - adenosine monophosphate
ANA - antinuclear antibody
Angio - angiography
AP - anteroposterior
ARDS - adult respiratory distress syndrome
ASD - atrial septal defect
ASO - anti-streptolysin O
AST - aspartate transaminase
AZT - zidovudine
BCG - bacille Calmette–Guérin
BP - blood pressure
BUN - blood urea nitrogen
CALLA - common acute lymphocytic leukemia antigen
CBC - complete blood count
CDC - Centers for Disease Control
CF - cystic fibrosis
CFTR - cystic fibrosis transmembrane conductance regulator
CHF - congestive heart failure
CK - creatine kinase
CNS - central nervous system
COPD - chronic obstructive pulmonary disease
CRP - C-reactive protein
CSF - cerebrospinal fluid
CT - computed tomography
CXR - chest x-ray
DIC - disseminated intravascular coagulation
DMD - Duchenne's muscular dystrophy
DTP - diphtheria/tetanus/pertussis
DTRs - deep tendon reflexes
DVT - deep venous thrombosis
EBV - Epstein–Barr virus
ECG - electrocardiography
Echo - echocardiography
ECMO - extracorporeal membrane oxygenation
EEG - electroencephalography
ELISA - enzyme-linked immunosorbent assay
EMG - electromyography
ESR - erythrocyte sedimentation rate
FEV - forced expiratory volume
FTA-ABS - fluorescent treponemal antibody absorption
FVC - forced vital capacity
GA - gestational age

Abbreviations - continued

G6PD - glucose-6-phosphate dehydrogenase
GI - gastrointestinal
Hb - hemoglobin
HGPRT - hypoxanthine-guanine phosphoribosyl transferase
HIV - human immunodeficiency virus
HLA - human leukocyte antigen
HPI - history of present illness
HR - heart rate
ID/CC - identification and chief complaint
IFA - immunofluorescent antibody
Ig - immunoglobulin
IM - intramuscular
INH - isoniazid
IVC - inferior vena cava
JRA - juvenile rheumatoid arthritis
JVP - jugular venous pressure
KUB - kidneys/ureter/bladder
LDH - lactate dehydrogenase
LFTs - liver function tests
LP - lumbar puncture
L/S - lecithin-to-sphingomyelin (ratio)
LV - left ventricular
LVH - left ventricular hypertrophy
Lytes - electrolytes
MI - myocardial infarction
MMR - measles/mumps/rubella
MR - magnetic resonance (imaging)
NG - nasogastric
NPO - nil per os (nothing by mouth)
NSAID - nonsteroidal anti-inflammatory drug
Nuc - nuclear medicine
PBS - peripheral blood smear
PCR - polymerase chain reaction
PDA - patent ductus arteriosus
PE - physical exam
PFTs - pulmonary function tests
PMI - point of maximal intensity
PPD - purified protein derivative
PT - prothrombin time
PTT - partial thromboplastin time
RBC - red blood cell
RF - rheumatoid factor
RPR - rapid plasma reagin
RR - respiratory rate
RSV - respiratory syncytial virus
RV - right ventricular
RVH - right ventricular hypertrophy
SBFT - small bowel follow-through

Abbreviations - continued

. . . .

SIDS - sudden infant death syndrome
TMP-SMX - trimethoprim-sulfamethoxazole
TSH - thyroid-stimulating hormone
UA - urinalysis
UGI - upper GI
URI - upper respiratory infection
US - ultrasound
VMA - vanillylmandelic acid
VS - vital signs
VSD - ventricular septal defect
vWF - von Willebrand factor
WBC - white blood cell
XR - x-ray

ID/CC	A 2-year-old **female** presents with **poor feeding** and **difficulty breathing.**
HPI	She was born in a small town in the Rocky Mountains (**high altitude** predisposes) and was delivered at 28 weeks' gestation (more common in **preterm** infants). On directed questioning, her mother recalls that she had a transitory skin rash during the first trimester of her pregnancy (**rubella** predisposes).
PE	VS: tachycardia; tachypnea. PE: **no cyanosis; bounding arterial pulses; wide pulse pressure;** hyperdynamic LV impulse displaced laterally; **continuous "machinery murmur"** noted at second and third left intercostal space lateral to sternal border.
Labs	ECG: left axis deviation; LVH.
Imaging	CXR: **increased pulmonary vascular markings;** enlarged left ventricle, left atrium, pulmonary arteries, and ascending aorta; the ductus arteriosus may show calcification. Echo: enlarged left atrium and ventricle. Angio: **increased oxygen saturation in the pulmonary artery** (diagnostic).
Pathogenesis	Failed closure of fetal communication between the pulmonary artery and aorta; commonly associated with maternal rubella and coxsackievirus infection, premature birth, and respiratory distress syndrome. The ductus normally closes as a result of increased oxygen tension during the first 48 hours of life (may take up to three weeks). The persistent communication between the descending aorta and pulmonary artery near the left subclavian artery increases pulmonary blood flow in systole and diastole, causing pulmonary congestion and LV overload.
Epidemiology	**Twice as common in females;** more common in infants born at high altitudes and in premature infants.
Management	In the presence of respiratory distress syndrome, **treat heart failure** (diuretics, digitalis) and anemia. **Indomethacin,** a prostaglandin E1 inhibitor, may stimulate ductus closure. **Surgery** consists of simple ligation (preferred), clipping, or division and may be considered in the absence of pulmonary hypertension. Administer **prophylactic antibiotics** with dental and

PATENT DUCTUS ARTERIOSUS

surgical procedures.

<table>
<tr><td>Complications</td><td>If left untreated, there is a high risk of left heart failure (most common), infective endocarditis, endarteritis, and Eisenmenger's syndrome (symptomatic pulmonary hypertension resulting from high pulmonary vascular flow; eventually leads to the development of a right-to-left shunt; manifests as right heart failure and cyanosis).</td></tr>
</table>

Associated Diseases

◘ **Atrial Septal Defect** The most common congenital heart disease in adults; acyanotic left-to-right shunt of left atrium into right atrium; presents with shortness of breath and systolic ejection murmur; fixed, wide split of S2; ECG shows right axis deviation; CXR shows increased pulmonary vascularity; treat by surgical repair; complications include paradoxic emboli, pulmonary hypertension, and Eisenmenger's syndrome (due to reversal of shunt).

◘ **Ventricular Septal Defect** An acyanotic cardiac malformation leading to left-to-right shunt; presents with dyspnea, parasternal heave, and pansystolic murmur; ECG reveals biventricular hypertrophy; CXR shows cardiomegaly; treat by surgical repair.

ID/CC	A 9-year-old girl presents with **shortness of breath** (= DYSPNEA) mostly while running or playing, coupled with lightheadedness and **easy fatigability** (due to decreased cardiac output).
HPI	Yesterday she complained of **severe chest pain** while skipping rope. She has no history of allergies, surgery, trauma, transfusions, hospitalizations, or major illnesses. Her vaccinations are up to date. The mother states that the child was born with **congenital rubella** (predisposing factor).
PE	VS: normal. PE: **raised JVP** with prominent "a" wave; presystolic liver pulsation (increased venous pressure); palpable **RV heave**; crescendo-decrescendo (diamond-shaped) **systolic ejection murmur** preceded by click in left second interspace (pulmonary area) radiating to neck; **soft P2 and widely split S2.**
Labs	CBC/Lytes: normal. ECG: right axis deviation; RV enlargement.
Imaging	**[A]** CXR: **poststenotic dilated pulmonary artery** (1); note the relative size of the aortic knob (2). Other findings include **diminished pulmonary vascular markings.** Echo: RV enlargement; dome-shaped valve. Angio: diagnostic; RVH with a transpulmonary gradient.
Pathogenesis	A **cyanotic** congenital heart disease that is **idiopathic,** although some viral infections have been implicated (congenital rubella is a predisposing factor). In the **neonatal** period, patients may present with **cyanosis** (right-to-left shunt through patent foramen ovale); mild disease may be asymptomatic. In moderate to severe disease there may be exertional dyspnea, hypoxic spells, squatting episodes (more typical of tetralogy of Fallot), and even ischemic chest pain. It may be isolated but is more commonly associated with a patent foramen ovale or with other cardiac defects, such as VSD, ASD, and PDA. May be **valvular, infundibular,** or combined. Associated with Noonan's syndrome and malignant intestinal carcinoid.
Epidemiology	Fifty percent of deaths occur within the first year of life unless a compensatory shunt (e.g., VSD, ASD, PDA)

PULMONARY STENOSIS

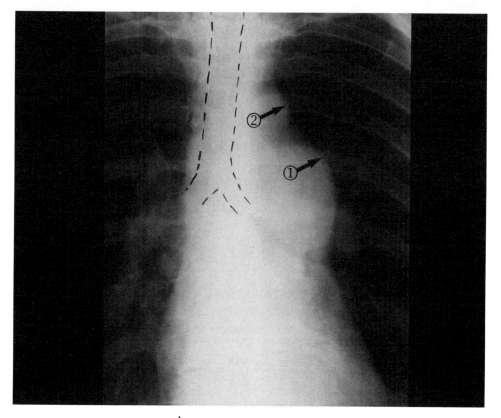

persists.

Management   **Prostaglandin E1** keeps the ductus arteriosus patent until surgery in neonates. **Balloon valvuloplasty** (mainly for isolated pulmonary stenosis) or surgical repair is required if the transpulmonary valve gradient exceeds 50 mmHg. **Emergent surgery** is indicated in acute right heart failure. RVH usually resolves after corrective surgery. Patients should be given antibiotic prophylaxis for **infective endocarditis** before dental and surgical procedures.

Complications   Complications include **cardiac failure** (most common), sudden death (most frequently in infancy), low cardiac output, growth retardation, hypoxic spells, and arrhythmias. Postoperative complications include recurrence (mainly if surgery was done early) and pulmonary insufficiency.

Associated Diseases   ◘ **Coarctation of the Aorta** Congenital stenosis of the aorta usually distal to the left subclavian artery; increased incidence in patients with Turner's syndrome; presents with weak and delayed femoral pulses, upper extremity hypertension, and systolic murmur heard loudest over the back; often asymptomatic but can cause claudication on exertion; CXR shows rib notching; chest CT documents the stenosis; treat with surgical resection of the stenosis with end-to-end anastomosis; complications include severe hypertension.

◘ **Tetralogy of Fallot** A cyanotic congenital defect with pulmonary stenosis, RVH, overriding aorta, and VSD; presents in young children with dyspnea on exertion, cyanotic "Tet spells," and clubbing of the fingers; polycythemia and hypoxemia; echo reveals cardiac defect; treat with surgical repair of cardiac defects.

ID/CC	A 3-year-old male presents with **failure to thrive.**
HPI	The patient has **not been gaining weight** normally and tends to **tire easily** while playing.
PE	No cyanosis; **displacement of PMI to left;** sternal lift; harsh, **holosystolic murmur** at left sternal border.
Labs	ABGs: normal. ECG: LVH; RVH.
Imaging	**[A]** CXR: enlarged heart and dilated pulmonary vessels (1). Echo: moderate defect in the interventricular septum. Angio: pulmonary-to-systemic blood flow ratio 1.5 to 1.0.
Pathogenesis	Can consist of isolated defects or of multiple anomalies. The opening is typically situated in the **membranous portion** of the septum; functional deficits depend on the size and status of the pulmonary vascular bed. The majority of patients have isolated large defects that are caught early in life. Two-dimensional echocardiography or color doppler examination can define the number and location of defects in the ventricular septum and detect other associated anomalies; hemodynamic and angiographic studies should be used to determine the status of the pulmonary vascular bed and to further assess the anatomy. Five to ten percent of patients with moderate VSD and left-to-right shunt develop RV outflow obstruction. Incompetence of the aortic valve is also observed in approximately 5% of patients. This results from insufficient cusp tissue or prolapse of the cusp through the interventricular defect. Aortic regurgitation then complicates and dominates the clinical course of these patients
Epidemiology	VSD is the **most common congenital heart disorder,** accounting for 26% of all congenital cardiac lesions.
Management	Patients with large VSDs (large left-to-right shunt) or pulmonary hypertension should undergo **surgical correction.** If corrected early, pulmonary vascular disease is easily reversed. Surgery typically is not recommended for patients with normal pulmonary arterial pressure.
Complications	VSD may close spontaneously (if small), but CHF and death may also result. Eisenmenger's syndrome may develop; aortic regurgitation and infective endocarditis

VENTRICULAR SEPTAL DEFECT

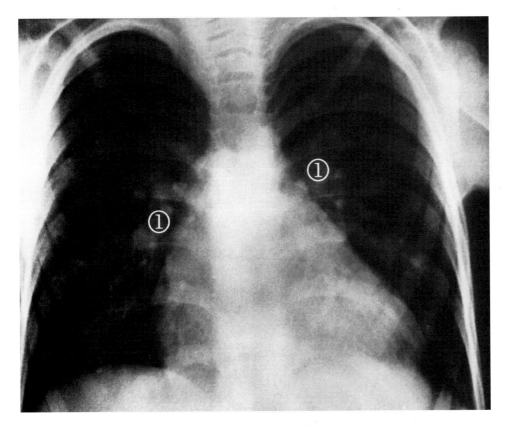

have also been observed.

◼ **Atrial Septal Defect** The most common congenital heart disease in adults; acyanotic left-to-right shunt of left atrium into right atrium; presents with shortness of breath and systolic ejection murmur; fixed, wide split of S2; ECG shows right axis deviation; CXR shows increased pulmonary vascularity; treat by surgical repair; complications include paradoxic emboli, pulmonary hypertension, and Eisenmenger's syndrome (due to reversal of shunt).

◼ **Patent Ductus Arteriosus** An acyanotic malformation connecting the aorta and left pulmonary artery; presents with a continuous "machinery murmur"; ECG shows left axis deviation; CXR reveals increased pulmonary blood flow; treat with surgical closure or indomethacin in neonates.

ID/CC	A newborn is seen by a neonatologist for **ambiguous genitalia.**
HPI	Her mother reports that the infant is **lethargic** and **lacks strength to suckle** (due to salt wasting). The parents are healthy with no relevant personal or family medical history.
PE	VS: no fever; hypotension; tachycardia. PE: well developed and nourished but **dehydrated; enlarged clitoris** and **fusion of labia majora.**
Labs	CBC: normal. Lytes: **hyponatremia; hyperkalemia. Increased serum 17-alpha-hydroxyprogesterone** and its metabolite **pregnanetriol** (can be detected prenatally); serum **androstenedione** and urinary **17-ketosteroids** elevated; elevated serum ACTH; low cortisol.
Imaging	XR-External Genitalia (with contrast media): **urogenital sinus.** CT-Abdomen: bilaterally enlarged adrenal glands.
Pathogenesis	Congenital adrenal hyperplasia (also known as **adrenogenital syndrome**) is an **autosomal-recessive** deficiency of metabolic enzymes (most commonly 21-hydroxylase) that results in the accumulation of substrate steroids (usually 17-alpha-hydroxyprogesterone) and a deficiency of normal adrenal steroids. It is usually recognized early by the characteristic genital ambiguity (due to virilization) and salt wasting. In older children, it may present as excessive muscularity, acne, excessive height, precocious sexual characteristics, and deep voice.
Epidemiology	**21-hydroxylase deficiency** is the most common form of congenital adrenal hyperplasia, accounting for 95% of cases. **Prenatal diagnosis** can be established in the first trimester by chorionic villous biopsy followed by HLA typing and in the second trimester by measurement of 17-OHP in amniotic fluid.
Management	Administer **cortisol** to suppress the hypersecretory adrenal gland and to prevent early epiphyseal closure and short stature in adults. If salt wasting is also present (half of cases), replace **mineralocorticoids** as well. Correction of external genitalia (in several operations) via **plastic surgery** can be done at a later date.

....

4.   **CONGENITAL ADRENAL HYPERPLASIA**

Complications	N/A
Associated Diseases	◘ **5-Alpha-Reductase Deficiency** An autosomal-recessive disorder of virilization; presents with microphallia, cryptorchidism, and hypospadias; decreased 5-alpha-dihydrotestosterone with normal testosterone level; treat with dihydrotestosterone.

CONGENITAL ADRENAL HYPERPLASIA

ID/CC	A 5-month-old **female** infant is seen for **sluggishness, edema,** and persistent **constipation.**
HPI	She appeared **normal at birth** except for mild **jaundice** that cleared somewhat but has not completely disappeared.
PE	VS: hypothermia; bradycardia. PE: mild jaundice; **dry skin; brittle hair; thick tongue; hoarseness;** hypertelorism; **flattened bridge of nose;** muscular **hypotonia; umbilical hernia;** short limbs; large anterior and posterior fontanelle.
Labs	CBC: anemia. **Low T4 and elevated TSH.**
Imaging	CXR: cardiomegaly. XR-Long Bones: delayed epiphyseal development (bone age); epiphyseal dysgenesis; beaking of T12 or L1 vertebrae; wormian bones.
Pathogenesis	Thyroid hormone deficiency (known as cretinism in children) may be primary or acquired. Most cases result from hypoplasia or aplasia or from embryologic maldescent of the thyroid. Other causes include hypothalamic and pituitary defects; deficiencies in iodine transport, concentration, organification, and coupling; failure of peripheral conversion of T4 to T3; peripheral resistance to thyroid hormone; defective thyroglobulin synthesis; and deficiency of iodide (= ENDEMIC CRETINISM). It may also be caused by exposure to phenylbutazone, iodides (present in expectorants), or sulfonamides or by excessive ingestion of cabbage by women during pregnancy.
Epidemiology	Affects approximately 1 in 4,000 newborns. Thyroid dysgenesis has a familial, summer-season, and **female predominance** and shows a higher incidence among Hispanics than among blacks or whites.
Management	A **newborn screening** test with TSH and T4 should be done in the first months of life to detect early hypothyroidism and to prevent mental retardation. Treatment involves the administration of **levothyroxine** with periodic TSH and T4 measurements.
Complications	**Mental retardation,** dwarfism, pathologic fractures, coxa vara, coxa plana, and iatrogenic hyperthyroidism.
Associated Diseases	❑ **Down's Syndrome** The most common chromosomal

disorder; due to trisomy 21; higher incidence in advancing maternal age; older patients with Down's syndrome are predisposed to Alzheimer's dementia; presents as developmentally retarded neonate with classic Down's facies (epicanthal folds, low-set ears, macroglossia), hypotonia, and simian crease; karyotype reveals trisomy 21; prenatal diagnosis is possible by chromosomal analysis of chorionic villous biopsy or amniocentesis and decreased levels of maternal serum alpha-fetoprotein levels; treatment consists of social service support; common complications include leukemia and heart disease.

ID/CC	A 15-month-old female appears **lethargic** after three days of persistent **vomiting** and **watery diarrhea** with no mucus or blood.
HPI	The mother states that the child has also had a mild **fever** and **does not have an appetite.** Her vaccinations are complete and up to date.
PE	VS: fever (38.2 C); **tachycardia** (HR 130); tachypnea (RR 21); hypotension. PE: **lethargic;** skin and mucous membranes are **pale, cold, and dry;** child cries but **no tears** are produced; **fontanelle is sunken;** poor skin turgor; abdomen slightly tender to palpation, but no masses or peritoneal signs; rectal exam reveals heme-negative stool (watery diarrhea).
Labs	CBC: **leukocytosis with lymphocyte predominance.** BUN and creatinine elevated; **stool shows no leukocytes** (nonbacterial diarrhea); stool culture and ova/parasites negative. ABGs: metabolic acidosis. Lytes: hypokalemia.
Imaging	CXR: normal. KUB: nonspecific small bowel loop dilatation.
Pathogenesis	The most common cause of gastroenteritis in children < 2 years is **rotavirus.** Infection is transmitted through feces (direct contact, contaminated food and drink).
Epidemiology	Rotavirus has a winter predominance.
Management	Most cases are treated with **oral rehydration;** for severe dehydration, IV rehydration is indicated. **Antibiotics** should be given for *Shigella* and invasive *E. coli* (TMP-SMX, ampicillin), amebiasis (metronidazole), cholera (tetracycline), and *Clostridium difficile* (vancomycin); symptoms of salmonellosis may be prolonged with antibiotics. **Anticholinergics are contraindicated** in children (prolong excretion of bacteria, virus particles, and exotoxins). Liquid diet low in lactose followed by soft diet.
Complications	The most common complication and cause of death **is fluid and electrolyte imbalance** (hypovolemia, metabolic acidosis, hypokalemia); other complications include septicemia (suspect in the presence of high fever, hypothermia, and lethargy without dehydration), acute renal failure (from acute hypovolemia), paralytic ileus, carbohydrate intolerance, pneumatosis intestinalis, and

GASTROENTERITIS

perforation with peritonitis and shock.

Associated Diseases ◙ **Cryptosporidiosis** Caused by *Cryptosporidium parvum;* presents as profuse, nonbloody, watery diarrhea, usually in AIDS patients; acid-fast staining demonstrates oocysts in fresh stool; treat with fluid and electrolyte repletion; AIDS patients should boil their water at home to prevent disease contraction.

◙ **Cholera** Caused by an exotoxin produced by *Vibrio cholerae,* activating intracellular adenylate cyclase; presents with profuse, watery diarrhea with "rice-water" appearance; stool exam reveals actively motile ("darting") gram-negative bacilli; treat with oral rehydration and electrolyte and glucose repletion, tetracycline; complications include progressive dehydration leading to hemodynamic collapse, particularly in children.

◙ **Giardiasis** The most common protozoal infection in children in the U.S.; transmitted through contaminated food or water; presents as an acute or chronic diarrhea (bulky, frothy, malodorous, greasy stools) associated with crampy abdominal pain and flatulence or may present as a malabsorption syndrome; binucleate, pear-shaped, flagellated trophozoites and cysts found in stool or duodenal fluid sample; treat with metronidazole.

◙ **Shigellosis** Due to *Shigella* enterotoxin, which activates adenylate cyclase; presents with nausea, vomiting, and dysentery; stool exam reveals leukocytes; culture isolates nonmotile *Shigella* bacterium; treat with rehydration and fluoroquinolones; complications include Reiter's syndrome and hemolytic-uremic syndrome (following *S. dysenteriae* infection).

ID/CC	A **2-year-old boy** presents with painless passage of **bright red blood per rectum** (= HEMATOCHEZIA).
HPI	The patient's medical history is unremarkable, and his vaccinations are up to date.
PE	VS: **tachycardia** (HR 156); no fever. PE: conjunctiva and mucous membranes **pale; abdomen tympanic and distended;** peristalsis increased; no palpable masses, hepatosplenomegaly, or peritoneal signs; heme-positive stool.
Labs	CBC: anemia; **leukocytosis** with **neutrophilia.**
Imaging	Nuc: technetium scan demonstrates **ectopic gastric mucosa** in the diverticulum. KUB: normal. **[A]** SBFT: another patient with a typical diverticulum. **[B]** Intraoperative visualization of a Meckel's diverticulum on the **antimesenteric border** of the intestine (vs. duplications and pseudodiverticula).
Pathogenesis	Due to **persistence of the vitelline duct** (normally closes during the fifth to seventh week of intrauterine life). In children, it presents as **painless rectal bleeding.** Meckel's diverticulum may be found in a hernia (= LITTRE'S HERNIA).
Epidemiology	The **most common congenital GI anomaly.** Predominantly affects males; characterized by the **rule of 2's:** affects 2% of population, 2 inches long, first 2 years of life, 2 feet from ileocecal valve, 2 types of epithelium (gastric and pancreatic).
Management	Achieve **fluid and electrolyte balance;** the definitive treatment is **surgical resection.** In the presence of peptic ulceration, the adjacent ileum is often involved and should be resected.
Complications	**Hemorrhage** (due to peptic ulceration; may be massive), **inflammation** (diverticulitis, appendicitis-like), **perforation, intussusception** (with intestinal obstruction), **umbilical drainage of ileal material** (omphaloenteric fistula, complete persistence of omphalomesenteric duct), **volvulus, foreign body obstruction,** and **intestinal obstruction** (fibrous remnants of vitelline artery to umbilicus); rarely, leiomyoma, carcinoid, and adenocarcinoma.

MECKEL'S DIVERTICULUM

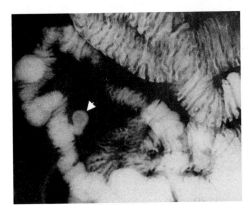 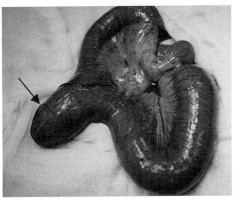

Associated Diseases

◻ **Inguinal Hernia** Protrusion of bowel through the abdominal wall due to an acquired defect in the floor of Hesselbach's triangle (borders are the inguinal ligament, inferior epigastric vessels, and lateral edge of rectus abdominis) (= DIRECT HERNIA) or through the inguinal canal (= INDIRECT HERNIA); presents with an asymptomatic lump in the groin that bulges with increased abdominal pressure (e.g., lifting heavy weight); can become painful; treatment is surgical reduction and repair of supporting tissue defect; complications include strangulation of bowel leading to bowel necrosis.

◻ **Hypertrophic Pyloric Stenosis** Congenital hypertrophy of the pyloric sphincter; common in first-born male neonates; usually presents at 2–6 weeks of age with projectile, nonbilious vomiting and an olive-like mass in the epigastrium; US shows pylorus muscle thickening; UGI reveals string sign; treat with surgical sphincterotomy.

◻ **Intestinal Malrotation with Volvulus** Congenital failure of the colon to rotate properly during embryogenesis, allowing the small bowel to twist within the mesentery due to lack of proper peritoneal attachment; presents with bilious vomiting, abdominal distention, and fever; abdominal XR shows air-fluid levels and lack of gas in the colon; CT or barium enema reveals the cecum to lie outside the right lower quadrant; treatment is emergent laparotomy with reduction of volvulus.

◻ **Necrotizing Enterocolitis** Idiopathic necrosis of bowel mucosa commonly seen in preterm newborns; presents with abdominal distention, bloody stools,

MECKEL'S DIVERTICULUM

bilious vomiting, and fever; abdominal XR reveals dilated loops of bowel and may show pathognomonic air within the bowel wall; treat with nasogastric tube bowel decompression, IV fluids, surgical laparotomy with bowel excision if disease progresses.

MECKEL'S DIVERTICULUM

ID/CC	A 10-year-old boy is admitted with **massive vomiting of bright red blood** (= HEMATEMESIS).
HPI	For two days, the child has been passing **black, tarry** (= MELENA), **foul-smelling stool.** His parents disclose that he has had similar episodes in the past, during which he was hospitalized and given multiple transfusions. Directed questioning also reveals that he received an umbilical exchange transfusion at birth.
PE	VS: tachycardia; orthostatic hypotension. PE: ill-looking and anxious; cold extremities; marked **pallor;** no icterus or clubbing; no signs of chronic liver disease; massive **splenomegaly.**
Labs	CBC: severe **normocytic anemia.** LFTs: normal. Coagulation profile normal; normal protein C and S levels; endoscopy shows presence of **actively bleeding varices.**
Imaging	US-Abdomen: splenomegaly with small reflective channels (suggestive of portal hypertension as cause). Doppler Studies: **extrahepatic obstruction of portal vein. [A]** Splenoportogram (now done rarely): massive collaterals with an enlarged splenic vein (1) and a completely obstructed (nonvisualized) portal vein; contrast directed to the esophageal (2) and gastric (3) varices and inferior mesenteric vein (retrograde flow). **[B]** UGI: multiple serpiginous filling defects in the esophagus typical of indentation by varices.
Pathogenesis	**Umbilical vein sepsis** due to umbilical catheterization is usually the cause of extrahepatic obstruction of the portal vein in neonates. Portal vein obstruction can also occur as a result of a tumor compressing the portal vein, but such an occurrence in childhood is exceedingly rare. **Recurrent variceal bleeding** and **splenomegaly** without evidence of liver dysfunction are the hallmarks of this disease.
Epidemiology	Portal vein thrombosis is the leading cause of portal hypertension in children without evidence of cirrhosis.
Management	Stabilize patients with immediate IV fluids and blood transfusions for acute bleeds; perform emergent upper GI endoscopy to confirm variceal bleed. **Scleropathy** and **portocaval shunting** can be used for long-term

PORTAL VEIN THROMBOSIS

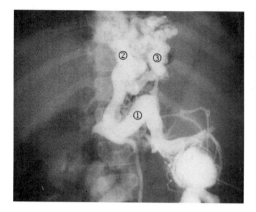

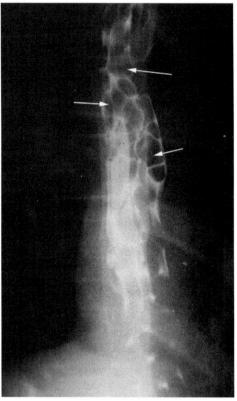

management of portal hypertension.

Complications   N/A

Associated Diseases   N/A

ID/CC	A 15-year-old girl presents with **jaundice,** spasmodic limb movements (= CHOREA), and **behavioral changes.**
HPI	She has been performing poorly in school, and her mother notes that she has become increasingly labile and confused over the past few months.
PE	VS: normal. PE: jaundice; hepatomegaly; **[A] Kayser–Fleischer ring** seen on slit-lamp exam.
Labs	Elevated serum copper; low ceruloplasmin. LFTs: elevated AST and ALT; elevated bilirubin. Prolonged PT/PTT (signs of hepatic dysfunction); liver biopsy demonstrates **elevated parenchymal copper.** UA: elevated 24-hour copper level.
Imaging	MR-Brain: cerebral atrophy with hypodensity of the caudate and putamen.
Pathogenesis	Wilson's disease is an **autosomal-recessive** disorder of copper metabolism secondary to a **deficiency of the copper-binding protein** (ceruloplasmin). This results in the abnormal accumulation of copper in the parenchymal cells of the liver, kidney, brain, and cornea. It most often manifests as **progressive hepatic dysfunction** that may be accompanied by **neuropsychiatric disorders.**
Epidemiology	Onset of disease is usually between the first and third decades of life.
Management	Chronic treatment with **copper-chelating agents** often halts the progress of the disease. **Liver transplantation** is indicated in cases of fulminant hepatic failure or progressive dysfunction despite chelation therapy.
Complications	Cirrhosis and hepatocellular carcinoma.
Associated Diseases	N/A

WILSON'S DISEASE

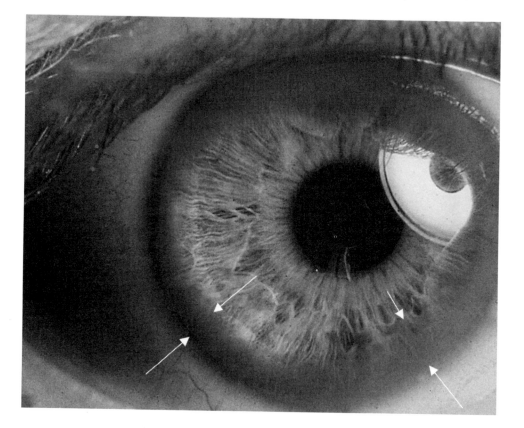

WILSON'S DISEASE

ID/CC	A 6-year-old boy presents with progressive **mental retardation, diminished visual acuity,** and **deformity of the bones of his chest.**
HPI	The boy exhibits marked **developmental delay.** Two years ago he developed a **DVT** of the left leg (due to hypercoagulability).
PE	VS: normal. PE: **fair skin;** tall and thin with **long limbs** and abnormally long fingers (= ARACHNODACTYLY); shuffling gait and mild **mental retardation** (due to recurrent cerebral thrombosis); fine hair and pectus carinatum; **glaucoma, cataracts,** and **lenticular dislocation** (= ECTOPIA LENTIS); **malar flush.**
Labs	CBC/Lytes: normal. **Increased plasma methionine and homocysteine.** UA: homocystinuria.
Imaging	XR: generalized **osteoporosis. [A]** XR-Spine: lumbar spine shows loss of bone density with vertebral collapse. **[B]** XR-Spine: normal lumbar spine for comparison.
Pathogenesis	An **autosomal-recessive** disorder involving hepatic **cystathionine beta-synthase deficiency.** Clinically characterized by **recurrent thromboembolic episodes** (hypercoagulable state due to increased platelet adhesiveness in the presence of elevated homocystine levels) as well as by lens dislocation (myopia may precede ectopia lentis), cataracts, mental retardation, seizures, astigmatism, glaucoma, and a marfanoid body type.
Epidemiology	Rare.
Management	Treatment is mainly supportive. In "decreased-affinity" cases, **high doses of pyridoxine and folic acid** may diminish mental retardation if started early in the course of the illness. In enzyme-deficient patients, dietary **restriction of methionine** and **cysteine supplementation** are necessary from infancy.
Complications	Cerebrovascular accidents, MI, arteriosclerotic heart disease, renal and pulmonary embolism, retinal detachment, and fractures.
Associated Diseases	◘ **Alport's Disease** An X-linked genetic connective tissue disease; presents with hematuria, deafness, renal failure, and lenticular dislocation; treat with corticosteroids for renal disease; consider renal

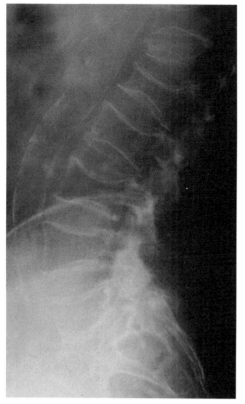 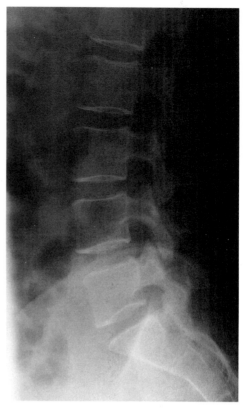

transplantation.

◻ **Ehlers–Danlos Syndrome** A group of genetic
disorders of collagen synthesis with variable inheritance;
presents with hyperelastic skin, hyperextensible joints,
and easy bruising; skin biopsy shows large irregular
collagen fibrils; treatment is supportive; patients are
prone to dissection and aneurysm of the great vessels.

ID/CC	A 10-year-old **mentally retarded boy** is brought to a physician by his parents because of bizarre, **self-destructive behavior.**
HPI	The boy frequently **bites his lips, fingers, and buccal mucosa.** Yesterday he attempted to put his hand in a fire. He has been **growth-retarded** since infancy. Last year he underwent surgery for bilateral **ureteral stones.** His maternal uncle had a similar disease and died of a self-inflicted head injury.
PE	VS: normal. PE: far below mental and physical standards appropriate for age; choreoathetoid movements of hands; lips and fingers have been bitten in multiple places; **spastic weakness and hyperreflexia** of lower limbs; tophi over extensor surfaces of elbows, knees, fingers, and toes.
Labs	Serum **uric acid levels markedly elevated (=** HYPERURICOSURIA). RBCs demonstrate **absence of enzyme hypoxanthine-guanine phosphoribosyltransferase (HGPRT).** UA: uric acid crystals.
Imaging	N/A
Pathogenesis	An **X-linked recessive disorder** seen only in males, it is caused by a severe deficiency of HGPRT, an enzyme that retrieves hypoxanthine and guanine through salvage pathways for utilization in nucleotide synthesis. In the absence of this enzyme, hypoxanthine and guanine can be catabolized only through xanthine to uric acid, causing hyperuricemia and markedly increased uric aciduria.
Epidemiology	N/A
Management	**Allopurinol** controls uric acid crystalluria and the tendency toward stone formation. It also prevents development of gouty arthritis (usually occurs after puberty). There is no specific therapy for neurologic symptoms.
Complications	N/A
Associated Diseases	◘ **von Gierke's Disease** An autosomal-recessive disease due to a deficiency of glucose-6-phosphatase; presents with fatigue and lightheadedness; hyperuricemia and

marked hypoglycemia; US shows hepatomegaly and enlarged kidneys; treat with frequent meals to prevent hypoglycemia.

LESCH-NYHAN SYNDROME

ID/CC	A 4-year-old male presents with **progressive mental retardation** and hyperactivity with purposeless movements.
HPI	The child **developed normally for the first 2–3 months**. He is **fairer** than his siblings and, unlike them, has blue eyes and blond hair (due to albinism). He did not undergo screening for any congenital disorder.
PE	Severely mentally retarded with **fair skin, blue eyes,** and characteristic **"mousy" or musty odor;** neurologic exam reveals hypertonicity with hyperactive DTRs.
Labs	Guthrie test (bacterial inhibition assay method) positive; **plasma phenylalanine elevated** (> 20 mg/dL); plasma tyrosine normal; elevated urinary phenylpyruvic and orth-hydroxyphenylacetic acid; tetrahydrobiopterin concentration normal. EEG: abnormal.
Imaging	N/A
Pathogenesis	An **autosomal-recessive** disease that is due to deficient or absent **phenylalanine hydroxylase,** resulting in toxic accumulation of phenylalanine and its metabolites. In maternal phenylketonuria, the persistent elevation of plasma phenylalanine concentration perfusing the heterozygous fetus during development increases the risk of mental retardation, heart defects, and prenatal growth delay.
Epidemiology	N/A
Management	Give **diet formulas low in phenylalanine** and monitor serum levels. Diet should also have **adequate amounts of tyrosine. Avoid aspartame** (Nutrasweet), which is broken down by the body into phenylalanine. **Neonatal screening** is essential in preventing the development of mental retardation in affected children.
Complications	N/A
Associated Diseases	N/A

PHENYLKETONURIA

ID/CC	A 10-year-old male presents with **recurrent fatigue,** anxiety, nausea, **lightheadedness,** and **sweating** (due to hypoglycemia) that are precipitated by short periods of **fasting** or **exercise.**
HPI	His mother states that his **symptoms are relieved by eating.** She adds that her son also has a **bleeding tendency** (due to platelet dysfunction). Occasionally he complains of severe **pain and swelling of his big toe** (due to gout).
PE	VS: normal. PE: pale; **obese** with **"doll's face";** no mental retardation; enlarged tongue (= MACROGLOSSIA); **low weight for age;** tendon xanthomas; purpuric spots on legs and arms; abdomen distended; **marked hepatomegaly;** no splenomegaly; soft **tophi** on elbows and ears.
Labs	CBC: normochromic anemia. **Elevated blood lactic and pyruvic acid** (= LACTIC ACIDOSIS); elevated serum uric acid (= HYPERURICEMIA); hypophosphatemia; **hypercholesterolemia; hypertriglyceridemia; severe fasting hypoglycemia** (glucose < 40 mg/dL); prolonged PT and bleeding time; **IV galactose/fructose does not raise blood glucose level** (not converted to glucose); IV glucagon is not followed by rise in blood glucose (= GLUCAGON TOLERANCE TEST); hepatic biopsy reveals fatty liver with increased deposition of glycogen (glycogen-lipid droplets) and absence of glucose-6-phosphatase.
Imaging	US: diffuse hepatomegaly; **kidneys enlarged bilaterally.**
Pathogenesis	An **autosomal-recessive** glycogen storage disease (type I) caused by a **deficiency** of **glucose-6-phosphatase,** it is characterized by failure to convert glucose-6-phosphate to glucose, with resulting deposition of glycogen in tissues. Von Gierke's disease presents at birth or in the first year of life and involves the liver, kidneys, and intestine. There is **no skeletal or cardiac muscle involvement (since this enzyme is normally absent here).**
Epidemiology	Von Gierke's disease is the **most common glycogen storage disease.**
Management	Give **frequent, small meals** (high in carbohydrates and

protein) to prevent hypoglycemia and ketosis; continuous overnight gastrointestinal tube feedings. Use probenecid and allopurinol for hyperuricemia and diazoxide for hypoglycemia. Portacaval shunts have not yielded encouraging results, with cirrhosis and hepatic encephalopathy as frequent complications. Abdominal US or CT should be performed every 6–12 months, as patients are at **risk for hepatoma.**

Complications

Cardiac failure, cyanosis, convulsions, coma, hepatic adenomas and carcinomas, and liver cirrhosis.

Associated Diseases

◘ **G6PD Deficiency** An X-linked genetic defect commonly seen in African Americans and patients of Mediterranean descent, predisposing to hemolysis due to drugs (sulfonamides, antimalarials, salicylates), fava beans, and infection; presents with acute-onset jaundice, fatigue, tachycardia, and arthralgias; anemia, decreased haptoglobin, reticulocytosis, and decreased levels of G6PD; treatment is cessation of exposure to inciting agent; transfusions may be necessary; IV fluids and alkalinization of urine to maintain renal function; severe hemolysis can lead to renal failure.

ID/CC	A **4-year-old white male** is brought to the pediatrician with **pallor, fever, and joint pain** of several days' duration. Today he had an episode of spontaneous nosebleed (= EPISTAXIS).
HPI	The child has been complaining of **fatigue** and **bone pain** on and off for the past two months and has also had **repeated URIs** over the past six months.
PE	VS: **fever** (38.3 C); tachycardia (HR 110). PE: mucous membranes and conjunctiva **pale;** epistaxis and gingival bleeding with minor pressure; **ecchymotic patches** on skin of legs and arms; generalized **lymphadenopathy;** **sternal tenderness** elicited on pressure; nontender **hepatosplenomegaly.**
Labs	CBC/PBS: normocytic, normochromic **anemia** (Hct 24); **leukopenia; lymphocytosis; thrombocytopenia** (40,000); **[A]** **numerous immature leukocytes (blast cells).** Increased serum LDH; increased serum uric acid (= HYPERURICEMIA); **CALLA** (CD10) **positive and terminal deoxytransferase positive** (marker of immature T and B lymphocytes; differentiates from nonlymphoblastic leukemia); bone marrow biopsy shows **sheets of malignant lymphoblasts** replacing normal marrow.
Imaging	CXR: mediastinal mass seen (common in T-cell-type ALL).
Pathogenesis	Malignant proliferation of bone marrow lymphocyte precursors (= LYMPHOBLASTS) with bone marrow infiltration. Radiation, alkylating agents, and benzene exposure are associated with increased risk. It is classified as types L1–L3 (L1 – childhood type; L2 – adult type; L3 – Burkitt's type) and may also be classified as B-cell (most common), T-cell, or small cell type. It is more commonly seen in **Down's syndrome,** in patients with chromosome 5 and 7 abnormalities, and in the twin siblings of patients with the disease.
Epidemiology	Acute lymphocytic leukemia (ALL) is the **most common pediatric malignancy,** followed by brain tumors. It comprises 80% of all childhood leukemias and has a male and white predominance. **Most childhood leukemias are acute.**

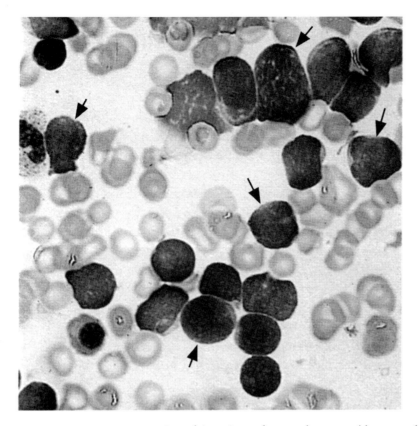

Management **Combination chemotherapy** (daunorubicin, vincristine, prednisone, and asparaginase) is used to induce remission (normal PBS and bone marrow morphology; clinically asymptomatic) and consolidation (= POSTREMISSION THERAPY). **Bone marrow transplantation** may also be considered. The vast majority of patients remit; most will not relapse. **Tumor lysis syndrome** after chemotherapy should be treated with allopurinol, urine alkalinization, hydration, and diuretics. Treat infection with antibiotics, anemia with transfusions, and thrombocytopenia with platelet concentrates. Given the risk of CNS disease, LP should be performed to rule out malignant involvement.

Complications Sepsis (*E. coli, Klebsiella, Pseudomonas, Candida*), meningitis, testicular and mediastinal involvement (more common with T-cell type), spontaneous bleeding (if platelet count < 20,000), and relapse. **FIRST AID 2** p. 191

Associated Diseases ☐ **Hodgkin's Lymphoma** Malignancy of lymphoid tissue, linked in some patients to EBV infection; presents with generalized lymphadenopathy, hepatosplenomegaly, fever, night sweats, and weight loss, or may present with asymptomatic adenopathy; chest and abdominal CT may reveal adenopathy and hepatosplenomegaly; lymph node biopsy shows Reed–Sternberg cells (necessary but not sufficient for diagnosis); treat with radiation therapy for local disease, allowing a nearly 90% five-year survival rate; add chemotherapy for metastatic disease.

▪ **Infectious Mononucleosis** A systemic EBV infection transmitted by respiratory droplets and saliva, primarily affecting teenagers and young adults; presents with sore throat, fever, lymphadenopathy, hepatomegaly, malaise, splenomegaly, and a maculopapular rash following ampicillin administration; atypical lymphocytes and positive heterophil antibody test; no treatment is required; the condition is self-limiting; avoid contact sports while splenomegaly is present; patients are at risk for splenic rupture in the convalescent phase.

▪ **Down's Syndrome** The most common chromosomal disorder; due to trisomy 21; higher incidence in advancing maternal age; older patients with Down's syndrome are predisposed to Alzheimer's dementia; presents as developmentally retarded neonate with classic Down's facies (epicanthal folds, low-set ears, macroglossia), hypotonia, and simian crease; karyotype reveals trisomy 21; prenatal diagnosis is possible by chromosomal analysis of chorionic villous biopsy or amniocentesis and decreased levels of maternal serum alpha-fetoprotein levels; treatment consists of social service support; common complications include leukemia and heart disease.

14. ACUTE LYMPHOCYTIC LEUKEMIA

ID/CC	A 7-year-old **male** is brought to an urgent-care clinic with an acutely **swollen and tender right knee** and a cut in his lip that has been **oozing blood** for the past day.
HPI	The child's **brother and maternal uncles died of bleeding complications,** and he has always had **easy bruising.** Yesterday he participated in a soccer game and fell several times.
PE	VS: normal. PE: small superficial laceration on inner aspect of lower lip that bleeds easily when touched with a cotton swab; knee swollen and warm to the touch with slight redness of skin; **multiple ecchymoses** on legs and arms.
Labs	CBC: mild normocytic **anemia. Normal bleeding time** (von Willebrand factor present); PT normal; **PTT prolonged; factor VIII:C level reduced;** factor VIII antigen normal.
Imaging	XR-Knee: soft tissue swelling with intra-articular fluid.
Pathogenesis	An **X-linked recessive** disorder associated with the absence or diminished activity of **factor VIII coagulant protein** (= FACTOR VIII:C). Factor VIII:C levels of < 1% are labeled as severe disease; levels between 1% and 5% indicate moderate disease; and levels > 5% are labeled as mild disease.
Epidemiology	Hemophilia A (factor VIII deficiency) accounts for 80% of cases; hemophilia B (factor IX deficiency, also known as Christmas disease; clinically indistinguishable from hemophilia A) accounts for 15% and hemophilia C (due to deficiency of factor XI) for 5%. The vast majority of patients have a **family history** of bleeding. Females are carriers and **males express the disease (X-linked recessive).**
Management	Parenteral **factor VIII concentrates** are the mainstay of therapy. Since the active life of factor VIII is not more than 24 hours, repeated doses are usually needed. **Desmopressin** IV or nasal spray may be used in mild to moderate cases by stimulating the body's production of endogenous factor VIII. Repeated **blood transfusions** are frequently required. Give ε-**aminocaproic acid** prior to dental work. Avoid aspirin and contact sports.
Complications	Intra-articular, intracranial, or intra-abdominal bleeding

as well as compartment syndrome and disabling joint disease may develop. Treated patients may develop inhibitors to factor VIII (which render exogenous factor VIII ineffective, causing refractory bleeding) and are at risk of acquiring HIV or hepatitis from multiple transfusions.

Associated Diseases

◘ **Hemophilia** An X-linked genetic defect of factor VIII (= HEMOPHILIA A) or of factor IX (= HEMOPHILIA B); presents in young children with hemorrhage, hemarthroses, and ecchymoses secondary to minor trauma; prolonged PTT and low factor VIII levels; treat with recombinant factor VIII or IX, transfusions as needed; complications include massive hemorrhage or acquisition of infections (e.g., HIV, hepatitis viruses) via blood and blood products.

◘ **Idiopathic Thrombocytopenic Purpura** Autoantibodies against platelets; affects children and young adults; often preceded by viral illness; presents with epistaxis and purpura; no palpable spleen; isolated thrombocytopenia and normal bone marrow with increased megakaryocytes; treat with high-dose prednisone, splenectomy.

◘ **von Willebrand's Disease** An inherited (mostly autosomal-dominant) disorder caused by a deficiency of von Willebrand factor (vWF); presents with episodic mucosal, GI, and dental bleeding and easy bruisability; increased bleeding time, prolonged PTT, and decreased ristocetin cofactor and factor VIII antigen; treat with avoidance of aspirin, use of desmopressin acetate, factor VIII concentrates that contain functional vWF and cryoprecipitate.

ID/CC	A 4-year-old boy is admitted with a **high-grade fever.**
HPI	His mother reveals that he has a history of **recurrent episodes of high-grade fever and mouth ulcers;** these episodes occur at intervals of 3–4 weeks. In between, the boy remains well.
PE	VS: tachycardia; high-grade **fever.** PE: multiple aphthous ulcers; cervical **lymphadenopathy; no hepatosplenomegaly or sternal tenderness.**
Labs	CBC: **leukopenia; absence of neutrophils;** neutrophil counts recover completely over following two weeks. Blood culture yields *S. aureus*.
Imaging	N/A
Pathogenesis	Cyclic neutropenia is characterized by **periodic wide fluctuations in neutrophil count.** The disorder is attributed to a regulatory defect of stem cells.
Epidemiology	The disease is rare and is generally detected in childhood. There is usually a positive **family history.**
Management	Administer **parenteral antibiotics;** give **G-CSF** to stimulate neutrophil production, shorten the duration of neutropenia, and help reduce the severity of symptoms and infections.
Complications	N/A
Associated Diseases	◨ **Chédiak–Higashi Syndrome** An autosomal-recessive defect of microtubule polymerization leading to impaired chemotaxis and phagocytosis; presents with recurrent pyogenic staphylococcal and streptococcal infections; decreased neutrophil count and large cytoplasmic granules; treat with antibiotics appropriate to infection. ◨ **Felty's Syndrome** Hypersplenism secondary to rheumatoid arthritis; presents with infections, purpura, and splenomegaly; neutropenia and thrombocytopenia; may have anemia; abdominal CT demonstrates enlarged spleen; treat the underlying rheumatoid arthritis; splenectomy may ameliorate disease.

ID/CC	A **5-year-old male** presents with **recurrent abdominal and joint pain.**
HPI	Yesterday his mother also noticed **black stools** (= MELENA; due to GI bleeding) and a **rash over his buttocks.** He has a **history of allergy** that includes atopic dermatitis in early infancy and intermittent asthma attacks. He suffered from a **URI one month ago.**
PE	VS: no fever; mild hypotension (BP 100/70); normal HR. PE: mild periorbital **edema; petechiae and palpable purpuric lesions** with **urticarial** features noted over extensor surfaces of **lower extremities** and **buttocks.**
Labs	CBC: mild leukocytosis; **normal platelets.** Elevated ESR. UA: **hematuria;** mild proteinuria. **Heme-positive stool; serum IgA increased;** kidney biopsy shows IgA and complement deposits; ANA negative.
Imaging	CXR/KUB: normal. US-Kidney: normal.
Pathogenesis	Henoch–Schönlein (= ANAPHYLACTOID) purpura is an **immune-mediated hypersensitivity vasculitis** characterized by inflammation and necrosis of small blood vessels (= LEUKOCYTOCLASTIC VASCULITIS). It is idiopathic with an allergic component and presents with a characteristic triad of **recurrent abdominal and joint pain, palpable purpura** over the buttocks and ankles, and **GI bleeding.**
Epidemiology	Seen more frequently in **males,** usually 2–5 years old, especially those with a history of **allergy** or **preceding URIs.**
Management	Treatment is often unnecessary. **Prednisone and analgesics** help ease abdominal pain. Improvement is usually seen within one month.
Complications	**Intussusception,** progressive **glomerulonephritis,** renal failure, and testicular torsion.
Associated Diseases	◨ **Hemolytic-Uremic Syndrome** Acute renal failure and microangiopathic hemolytic anemia, usually associated with bacterial (*E. coli, Shigella*) infection in children or following cancer chemotherapy (mitomycin); presents with fever, malaise, hypotension, ecchymoses, periorbital edema, and oliguria; schistocytes seen on PBS;

no evidence of DIC (normal PT, PTT, fibrinogen); thrombocytopenia and elevated BUN and creatinine; treat with plasmapheresis, IV fluids and pressors as needed to prevent acute renal failure and hemodynamic compromise.

◘ Idiopathic Thrombocytopenic Purpura

Autoantibodies against platelets; affects children and young adults; often preceded by viral illness; presents with epistaxis and purpura; no palpable spleen; isolated thrombocytopenia and normal bone marrow with increased megakaryocytes; treat with high-dose prednisone, splenectomy.

◘ Thrombotic Thrombocytopenic Purpura An

idiopathic disease found in pregnant and HIV-positive patients and after exposure to antibiotics or estrogens; presents with episodic altered mental status, fever, renal dysfunction, petechiae over the chest and extremities, and fever; anemia, schistocytes on smear, low platelet count, and absent haptoglobin; treat with plasmapheresis.

ID/CC	A 4-year-old girl is seen for **easy bruising** and a generalized nonpruritic **rash** of three days' duration.
HPI	She is a healthy child except for a history of easy bruising and frequent nosebleeds that started after a **URI two weeks ago.** She is not taking any medications.
PE	VS: normal. PE: **hemorrhagic bullae** on buccal mucosa; mucosal petechiae in conjunctiva and mouth; **[A]** **generalized small, red, flat subcutaneous macules** that do not blanch on pressure (= PETECHIAL RASH), distributed primarily on **pressure points;** no splenomegaly.
Labs	CBC/PBS: slight anemia (Hb 10.2); **platelet count decreased** with giant platelets (= MEGATHROMBOCYTES). **PT/PTT normal;** bone marrow shows **normal megakaryocytes** (indicating peripheral bone marrow destruction); **anti-platelet IgG antibodies** present.
Imaging	CXR/KUB: normal.
Pathogenesis	An idiopathic condition in which antibodies are formed against one's own platelets (resulting in splenic destruction and thrombocytopenia with bleeding tendency); it generally occurs 2–3 weeks after an infection (usually a URI) and is usually associated with a history of nasal, gum, or urinary bleeding. The rash is petechial, and platelets are characteristically low with prolonged bleeding time. The childhood form is usually acute and self-limited; the adult form is chronic.
Epidemiology	Acute, severe thrombocytopenia following a viral URI or exanthem is seen most commonly among children. The chronic form is common among adults, particularly women (between 20 and 40 years), who outnumber men by a ratio of 3 to 1.
Management	The disease is **usually self-limited** with resolution of petechiae within 1–2 weeks and normalization of platelet count within six months. Treat more severe cases (platelets < 20,000) with **steroids** or **platelet concentrates. Splenectomy** should be performed if the disease is steroid resistant after 6–12 months. IV high-dose **gamma globulin** and **azathioprine** may also

IDIOPATHIC THROMBOCYTOPENIC PURPURA

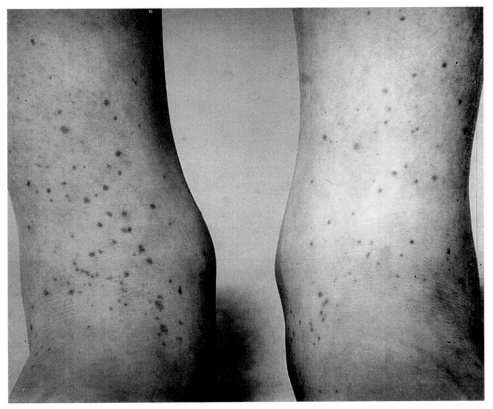

elevate platelet counts. Avoid aspirin.

Complications   Bleeding into tissue, head, chest, or abdomen following minor trauma.

Associated Diseases   ◘ **Thrombotic Thrombocytopenic Purpura** An idiopathic disease found in pregnant and HIV-positive patients and after exposure to antibiotics or estrogens; presents with episodic altered mental status, fever, renal dysfunction, petechiae over the chest and extremities, and fever; anemia, schistocytes on smear, low platelet count, and absent haptoglobin; treat with plasmapheresis.

◘ **Henoch–Schönlein Purpura** A self-limiting purpuric vasculitis due to immune complex deposition; common in children; presents with a palpable puerperal rash on the buttocks and legs, abdominal pain, fever, and arthralgia; renal biopsy reveals segmental glomerulonephritis with crescents and mesangial IgA deposition; treatment is not required; complications include very rare progression to glomerulonephritis.

ID/CC	A 4-year-old **black** male presents with **swelling of the hands and feet** (= DACTYLITIS), fever, headache, and a feeling of heaviness in the abdomen (splenomegaly).
HPI	The child has had **recurrent abdominal and joint pain** (due to ischemia) and recently noted an **increased appetite for salt.** He has also been wetting his bed (= ENURESIS) recently. The child's cousin also suffers from a blood disorder.
PE	VS: **fever** (38.3 C). PE: **in pain; pallor** of conjunctiva, skin, and mucous membranes (due to anemia); mild icterus (due to hemolysis); hypoxic spots with neovascularization on retina; throat hyperemic; regular rate and rhythm with no murmurs; lungs clear; **splenomegaly;** skin over metacarpals and metatarsals is warm to touch; **joints tender.**
Labs	CBC/PBS: **[A]** **sickle-shaped erythrocytes; anemia;** Howell–Jolly bodies and target cells; **reticulocytosis;** leukocytosis; thrombocytosis. LFTs: hyperbilirubinemia (unconjugated); increased LDH. Absent haptoglobin; sickling of RBCs when exposed to sodium metabisulfite (screening); electrophoresis shows **predominantly HbS,** some HbF, and no HbA (= ADULT). UA: microscopic hematuria.
Imaging	XR-Hands and Feet: soft tissue swelling with radiolucent areas (bone necrosis).
Pathogenesis	An **autosomal-recessive hemoglobinopathy** (HbS) due to a mutation in the gene coding for the beta chain of hemoglobin **(glutamic acid for valine at position 6).**
Epidemiology	Incidence is **1 in 400 African Americans** (most common hemoglobinopathy in blacks); 7% of black Americans have the sickle cell trait. **Dactylitis** is the most frequent initial manifestation. Onset is at 6–12 months, when HbF (which confers protection against sickling) disappears.
Management	Treat crises with **pain control** (avoid meperidine owing to risk of normeperidine accumulation and seizures) and **aggressive hydration.** Transfuse if more anemic than baseline (sickle cell patients are chronically anemic). Treat infections. Laser therapy for retinopathy. Other measures include vaccination against *H. influenzae* B,

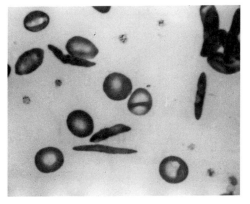

hepatitis, and pneumococcus as well as penicillin prophylaxis. Administer hydroxyurea (may increase HbF level). Oxygen, folic acid, exchange transfusion (for stroke, preoperatively, or for priapism), and marrow transplant may be given in severe cases.

Complications **Autosplenectomy** (due to repeated thrombosis), which increases the risk of bacterial infections by encapsulated organisms (e.g., meningitis, pneumonia, and *Salmonella* **osteomyelitis**), bone infarction with necrosis (RBCs sickling in the sinusoids), anesthetic complications, zinc deficiency, chronic leg ulcers, aseptic necrosis of the femoral head, retinal infarcts, and renal papillary necrosis.

Associated Diseases ◻ **G6PD Deficiency** An X-linked genetic defect commonly seen in African Americans and patients of Mediterranean descent, predisposing to hemolysis due to drugs (sulfonamides, antimalarials, salicylates), fava beans, and infection; presents with acute-onset jaundice, fatigue, tachycardia, and arthralgias; anemia, decreased haptoglobin, reticulocytosis, and decreased levels of G6PD; treatment is cessation of exposure to inciting agent; transfusions may be necessary; IV fluids and alkalinization of urine to maintain renal function; severe hemolysis can lead to renal failure.

◻ **Osteomyelitis** A pyogenic bone infection most commonly caused by *S. aureus;* presents with pain, swelling, warmth, redness, and immobility of joint; elevated ESR; MR reveals new osteoblastic periosteal bone formation (= INVOLUCRUM) with trapping of necrotic bone (= SEQUESTRUM); treat with surgical debridement and at least six weeks of IV antibiotics.

◻ **Thalassemia** An inherited defect of the alpha or beta chain of hemoglobin; common in African (beta defects), Southeast Asian (alpha defect), and Mediterranean populations; presents with chronic anemia of variable severity; target cells seen on blood smear; increased fetal hemoglobin and increased HbA2 on electrophoresis; treat with blood transfusions, folic acid supplements, and iron chelation therapy due to risk of iron overload from chronic transfusion.

ID/CC	A 13-year-old girl presents with **prolonged (> 7 days) and excessive (> 50 mL) menses** that began with menarche two weeks ago.
HPI	She has a history of **recurrent nosebleeds** (= EPISTAXIS) and **prolonged bleeding** from scratches and cuts. Her father also has a bleeding problem.
PE	VS: normal. PE: nasal mucosa bleeds excessively with nasal speculum examination; **petechial lesions** seen on arms, legs, and back of chest; bright red blood with clots in vaginal vault.
Labs	CBC: anemia; normal platelets. Normal PT; **prolonged bleeding time;** moderately **prolonged aPTT** (intrinsic system); reduced factor VIII by quantitative assay; low von Willebrand factor (vWF); ristocetin cofactor assay shows decreased platelet aggregation.
Imaging	CXR/KUB: normal.
Pathogenesis	Most commonly inherited as an **autosomal-dominant** bleeding disorder characterized by **impaired platelet aggregation induced by ristocetin;** vWF is secreted by endothelial cells and binds platelet surface receptor Gp1b, bridging platelet to subendothelial matrix to form the initial hemostatic plug. Deficient or dysfunctional vWF therefore results in prolonged bleeding time. Since vWF also serves as a plasma carrier for factor VIII, its deficiency is accompanied by reduced factor VIII activity.
Epidemiology	The **most common congenital disorder of hemostasis** (more common than hemophilia); seen in both sexes.
Management	**Avoid aspirin,** provide reassurance, and **administer factor VIII concentrate.** Desmopressin is used for bleeding prophylaxis before surgical procedures (including dental), complemented by tranexamic acid (antifibrinolytic) to prevent bleeding. Desmopressin should not be given in von Willebrand's disease type IIb.
Complications	N/A
Associated Diseases	◪ **Bernard–Soulier** A genetic defect in a receptor protein causing platelet dysfunction; presents with purpura and excessive bleeding in childhood; giant platelets seen on peripheral blood smear; no effective

treatment.

◼ **Hemophilia** An X-linked genetic defect of factor VIII (= HEMOPHILIA A) or of factor IX (= HEMOPHILIA B); presents in young children with hemorrhage, hemarthroses, and ecchymoses secondary to minor trauma; prolonged PTT and low factor VIII levels; treat with recombinant factor VIII or IX, transfusions as needed; complications include massive hemorrhage or acquisition of infections (e.g., HIV, hepatitis viruses) via blood and blood products.

ID/CC	A 7-year-old **male** is admitted to the hospital for evaluation of a **suspected immune deficiency.**
HPI	During infancy, the child had **atopic dermatitis.** His mother adds that he has had **recurrent skin, ear, and chest infections.** He also has recurrent episodes of **epistaxis.**
PE	VS: normal. PE: **eczematous skin rash** over flexor skin surfaces; **dry, lichenified skin lesions** over face, arms, and extremities; **bilateral otitis media.**
Labs	CBC: anemia; **thrombocytopenia.** Normal levels of IgG; **high levels of IgE and IgA; reduced levels of IgM;** anergic to bacterial and fungal antigens; **nitroblue tetrazolium test normal.**
Imaging	CXR: normal.
Pathogenesis	Wiskott–Aldrich syndrome is characterized by **eczema, thrombocytopenia, and increased susceptibility to infection** (mainly encapsulated organisms). The gene for Wiskott–Aldrich syndrome has been mapped to the X chromosome. The syndrome is associated with secondary malignancies, especially non-Hodgkin's lymphoma.
Epidemiology	An **X-linked recessive** disease seen predominantly in males.
Management	Requires **bone marrow transplantation** after administering irradiation or busulfan and antilymphocyte serum to destroy residual lymphocytes. Patients have subsequently shown normal immune and platelet function.
Complications	Infection and malignancy.
Associated Diseases	◻ **Atopic Dermatitis** An idiopathic, chronic, IgE-mediated skin inflammation; presents with intense pruritus, lichenification secondary to scratching, erythema, and scaling; treat with topical corticosteroids, hydrating creams, and removal of potential allergens; complications include secondary infection.
	◻ **Henoch–Schönlein Purpura** A self-limiting purpuric vasculitis due to immune complex deposition; common in children; presents with a palpable puerperal rash on

the buttocks and legs, abdominal pain, fever, and arthralgia; renal biopsy reveals segmental glomerulonephritis with crescents and mesangial IgA deposition; treatment is not required; complications include very rare progression to glomerulonephritis.

WISKOTT–ALDRICH SYNDROME

ID/CC	A **1-year-old** male presents with **respiratory distress, coughing** (dry and hacking; sometimes paroxysmal), **and wheezing** of four hours' duration.
HPI	Immunizations are up to date. Others in his day-care center have had similar symptoms.
PE	VS: **tachycardia; marked tachypnea; low-grade fever.** PE: in acute distress; **dyspnea** noted (nasal flaring and use of accessory muscles of respiration); no cyanosis (vs. pertussis and epiglottitis); no conjunctivitis (vs. chlamydial pneumonia); no drooling (vs. epiglottitis); **audible expiratory wheezes;** no inspiratory stridor (vs. croup); **rales, crackles, and rhonchi** heard on auscultation.
Labs	CBC: leukocytosis with **lymphocytosis.** ABGs: **hypoxemia.** Sputum culture reveals **normal flora;** pertussis culture negative; **viral culture RSV positive** (gold standard); nasopharyngeal washings (ELISA or immunofluorescence) RSV positive.
Imaging	CXR: **hyperinflation** with air trapping, flattened diaphragms, increased bronchovascular markings, peribronchial cuffing, segmental **atelectasis,** and **interstitial infiltrates.**
Pathogenesis	A lower respiratory tract infection of viral origin, usually **RSV,** in which epithelial necrosis, increased mucus, and edema lead to obstruction and atelectasis. At increased risk are immune-compromised patients, premature infants, and those with congenital heart diseases.
Epidemiology	Usually **symptomatic in children 6–12 months** of age; less symptomatic in children > 2 years. Occurs in yearly epidemics, primarily in **winter** and **spring.**
Management	Management is primarily **supportive:** nutrition (IV or NG tube), humidified oxygen, nebulized beta-2 agonists, and ventilatory support. Amantadine should be given in the presence of influenza virus; prophylactic monoclonal antibody to RSV can be given in the presence of pulmonary disease, epidemics, or prematurity. Most patients recover in four days.
Complications	Bacterial superinfection (otitis media, bronchitis, bronchopneumonia), cyanosis, apneic spells, respiratory

insufficiency, fatigue, and dehydration (from poor feeding).

Associated Diseases

◘ **Asthma** Bronchial constriction due to increased smooth muscle tone (hyperreactivity), mucosal edema (inflammation), and inspissated mucus plugs; presents with reversible episodic bronchoconstriction leading to acute dyspnea, hypoxia, and respiratory failure; increase in peak expiratory flow after administration of bronchodilator; treat acutely with albuterol and ipratropium inhalers; add corticosteroids if severe attack; intubate if necessary; use bronchodilators with or without inhaled corticosteroids for chronic treatment.

◘ **Chlamydial Pneumonia** Caused by *Chlamydia pneumoniae;* presents with productive cough and dyspnea; CXR shows lower lobe interstitial infiltrate; treat with erythromycin.

◘ **Croup** Caused by parainfluenza virus; spread by respiratory droplets; presents with sore throat and inspiratory stridor; throat and nasal swabs isolate the causative virus; neck XR may show subglottic narrowing ("steeple sign"); treat with oxygen, bronchodilators, racemic epinephrine.

◘ **Epiglottitis** Commonly caused by *H. influenzae;* presents with fever, hoarseness, odynophagia, drooling, and characteristic "sniffing-dog" position; cultures of throat swab and blood are positive; XR of the neck shows marked edema of the epiglottis (= "THUMBS UP" SIGN); treat with IV cefuroxime and airway maintenance; throat exam may precipitate laryngospasm and complete airway obstruction.

◘ **Pertussis** Caused by a toxin produced by *Bordetella pertussis;* presents in three stages: a catarrhal stage with sneezing and nocturnal cough, a paroxysmal stage with frequent productive "whooping cough" with vomiting, and a slow convalescent stage; nasal swab culture reveals organism; treat with oxygen as needed; place the patient in strict respiratory isolation; erythromycin to decrease duration of carrier state.

ID/CC	A 6-year-old male presents with an **inability to hear.**
HPI	The child's mother is an immigrant who received **no prenatal care.** At birth he appeared normal. The mother states that the child also appears **developmentally delayed** with speech problems. He has exhibited photophobia and increased lacrimation.
PE	VS: normal. PE: **saddlenose** and **poorly developed maxilla; centrally notched** (due to defectively formed enamel), **widely spaced, small, peg-shaped upper incisors** (= HUTCHINSON'S TEETH); thickening of anterior tibial area **(saber shins);** optic atrophy and exudative vascularization of cornea.
Labs	**Positive RPR** and FTA-ABS.
Imaging	XR-Long Bones: osseous abnormalities include luetic metaphysitis, diaphysitis, and periostitis; symmetric destruction of the medial portion of the proximal tibial metaphysis (= WIMBERGER'S SIGN) is pathognomonic; diffuse anterior thickening of the upper half of the tibial cortex (= SABER TIBIA).
Pathogenesis	Congenital syphilis is caused by *Treponema pallidum,* a spirochete that may cross the placenta at any stage of pregnancy. Adequate treatment prior to gestational week 16 generally prevents fetal sequelae. Prior to this time, the fetal immune system is incompetent, suggesting that the damage results from the fetal immune response to *T. pallidum* rather than from direct toxicity. The most characteristic **triad** of late congenital syphilis consists of **interstitial keratitis, Hutchinson's teeth,** and **eighth nerve deafness.** Since maternal-fetal transmission is rare before the fifth month, syphilis is an uncommon cause of abortion.
Epidemiology	One in 10,000 live newborn infants is infected. With untreated early maternal syphilis, the rate of transmission is 75%–90%. With maternal infection of two years or more, the rate of transmission is 35%.
Management	Penicillin G is the only recommended therapy. **Empiric treatment** is indicated in neonates who may not have follow-up and whose status is equivocal. All women should receive **screening** at their first prenatal visit; women at high risk should receive repeat screening in

CONGENITAL SYPHILIS

their third trimester and at delivery.

Complications Stillbirth and mental retardation.

Associated Diseases ◘ **Congenital Toxoplasmosis** Transplacental transmission; primary infection is derived from consumption of raw meat or contact with cat feces; presents with neonatal hydrocephalus, retardation, and seizures; MR or CT reveals intracranial ring-enhancing, calcified lesions; treat with pyrimethamine and sulfadiazine; avoid exposure.

◘ **HIV Transmission in Pregnancy** Vertical transmission of HIV most commonly occurring in the third trimester or during birth; presents with acute retroviral syndrome (e.g., fever, malaise, adenopathy) in the first months of life; PCR detection of HIV from newborn's blood; prevention is the treatment; give AZT to the mother during the third trimester or at least during labor, markedly diminishing the rate of transmission (from 24% to 8%).

ID/CC	A **newborn baby** is seen for an **extensive maculopapular rash** and **fever**.
HPI	His mother received no prenatal care and lives alone with a **pet cat**. She did not report any rashes or illnesses during pregnancy.
PE	VS: tachycardia; moderate tachypnea; fever. PE: **small for gestational age;** microcephalic with **extensive maculopapular rash** (spares soles, palms, and scalp); **chorioretinitis** with yellow-white, fluffy exudates clustered in posterior pole; **hepatosplenomegaly.**
Labs	CBC: thrombocytopenia. IFA for **IgM antibodies positive;** ELISA for IgM positive; **ToRCH test** on maternal serum (To = *Toxoplasma,* R = rubella, C = CMV, H = herpes zoster) also positive for *Toxoplasma* infection; serologic tests for syphilis, CMV, HIV, and rubella negative in neonate.
Imaging	XR-Skull: **calcifications.** CT-Head: **diffuse cerebral calcification** (vs. periventricular calcification seen in CMV inclusion disease).
Pathogenesis	*Toxoplasma gondii,* **an obligate intracellular protozoan** parasite, is the causative agent in toxoplasmosis. Infection via the oral route is caused by the ingestion of *T. gondii* cysts in undercooked food or by the ingestion of *T. gondii* oocysts, which are found in **cat feces.** If the **initial infection occurs during pregnancy,** parasitemia can cause **transplacental infection** of the fetus. Mothers with **chronic or latent toxoplasmosis** acquired before pregnancy **do not transmit** the infection to their children.
Epidemiology	Only half of all infants with congenital toxoplasmosis show clinical evidence of infection.
Management	**Pyrimethamine and sulfadiazine** used in combination for afflicted infants; folinic acid to prevent bone marrow suppression. Spiramycin should be started immediately for pregnant women. **Therapeutic abortion** might be considered if the infection is acquired early in pregnancy. Prevention is key and involves **avoidance** by minimizing contact with **cat feces** (not changing the cat litter) and not eating **undercooked meat.**

Complications	N/A
Associated Diseases	◘ **HIV Transmission in Pregnancy** Vertical transmission of HIV most commonly occurring in the third trimester or during birth; presents with acute retroviral syndrome (e.g., fever, malaise, adenopathy) in the first months of life; PCR detection of HIV from newborn's blood; prevention is the treatment; give AZT to the mother during the third trimester or at least during labor, markedly diminishing the rate of transmission (from 24% to 8%).

ID/CC	A 9-month-old female is seen after the development of a **brassy, barking cough.**
HPI	The patient is otherwise healthy and is up to date with her vaccinations. She has also been suffering from a **URI** of six days' duration, which is characterized by fever, malaise, rhinorrhea, and a runny nose.
PE	VS: low-grade fever (38.2 C). PE: restless and in **respiratory distress** with suprasternal and intercostal retractions; intermittent **inspiratory stridor; hoarse, barking cough;** diminished breath sounds bilaterally and scattered rales.
Labs	CBC: normal.
Imaging	XR-Neck: on AP view, **steeple sign** (subglottic narrowing, vs. "thumbprint sign" on lateral view in epiglottitis).
Pathogenesis	Caused primarily by the **parainfluenza virus.** Other offenders include influenza virus, adenovirus, and RSV (although the latter typically produces bronchiolitis).
Epidemiology	Most commonly occurs in patients between the ages of six months and six years, with a male predominance. Seen more frequently in **fall** and **winter** (during change from warm to cold weather).
Management	Mild cases can be **managed supportively** on an outpatient basis. Mist therapy, oxygen, **racemic epinephrine,** acetaminophen, and corticosteroids (if severe) may be useful. Hospitalize if there is stridor at rest.
Complications	Respiratory failure, dehydration due to inability to feed, and pneumonia. **FIRST AID 2** p. 291
Associated Diseases	◻ **Bronchiolitis** Most commonly caused by RSV in infants; presents with wheezing, nasal flaring, rhonchi, and congestion; lymphocytosis and hypoxemia; positive culture of throat swab; CXR shows hyperinflation and atelectasis; treat with humidified oxygen and fluid management, ribavirin for children with underlying heart or lung disease. ◻ **Epiglottitis** Commonly caused by *H. influenzae*; presents with fever, hoarseness, odynophagia, drooling,

and characteristic "sniffing-dog" position; cultures of throat swab and blood are positive; XR of the neck shows marked edema of the epiglottis (= "THUMBS UP" SIGN); treat with IV cefuroxime and airway maintenance; throat exam may precipitate laryngospasm and complete airway obstruction.

CROUP

ID/CC	An 8-year-old male is seen for a low-grade fever and **facial rash.**
HPI	His brother had a similar rash a few days ago. He has not had hematuria (rule out poststreptococcal glomerulonephritis).
PE	VS: low-grade fever (38 C). PE: **multiple vesicles and pustules** over the face and behind the ears measuring about 5 mm in diameter; lesions coalesce at places and are covered by a **honey-colored crust;** preauricular and **superficial cervical lymphadenopathy.**
Labs	Gram stain of exudate from rash shows **gram-positive cocci in chains;** culture yields **group A beta-hemolytic streptococci.** UA: normal.
Imaging	N/A
Pathogenesis	The causative agent is most commonly **group A streptococci** (90% *S. pyogenes*; *S. aureus* causes bullous impetigo). Impetigo is the most common streptococcal skin infection that **predisposes to glomerulonephritis.**
Epidemiology	Impetigo is **highly communicable** and occurs predominantly among preschoolers. Outbreaks of pyoderma-associated nephritis can occur in families or may spread in communities. The frequency of acute glomerulonephritis following infection caused by a known nephritogenic strain is 10%–15%. The nephritogenic strains associated with pyoderma (types 49, 52, 53, 55–57, and 61) differ from the pharyngitis-associated nephritogenic strains (types 1, 4, 12, and 25).
Management	**Oral penicillin** is the drug of choice for impetigo and ecthyma. **Erythromycin** is used in penicillin-allergic patients.
Complications	Pyoderma-associated nephritis.
Associated Diseases	◨ **Erysipelas** Infection, commonly on the face, by *Streptococcus pyogenes;* presents with the characteristic bright red, raised macule with well-demarcated borders, fever, and pain; treat with penicillin.

ID/CC	A 4-month-old infant is seen for **difficulty breast feeding.**
HPI	The mother also noticed that the child has been **constipated** for the past few weeks. The infant has **regularly been given honey** that his grandmother brought him.
PE	VS: tachycardia; tachypnea; normal BP. PE: **hypotonic;** breathing appears shallow and labored (**diaphragm weakness); motor development retarded;** poor sucking and rooting reflex; weight and height normal for age; no hepatosplenomegaly; **ptosis; pupils dilated** and **sluggishly reacting to light.**
Labs	EMG: characteristic pattern of **brief, small, abundant motor-unit action potentials** noted. Normal nerve conduction; stool culture yields *Clostridium botulinum* growth and toxin detected in feces; *C. botulinum* toxin present in blood. LP: **CSF normal.**
Imaging	N/A
Pathogenesis	The disease in infants is thought to be caused by **colonization** of the intestine and subsequent release of toxin by *C. botulinum*, with later **absorption of the toxin. Honey** has been implicated in at least one-third of cases.
Epidemiology	Infant botulism has been reported worldwide. Most cases occur in California, where spores are present in soil and on many vegetables.
Management	**Ventilatory** and **nutritional support** are the mainstays of treatment. **Polyvalent autotoxin** (made in horses) should be given after sensitivity testing. Avoid consumption of honey in children < 1 year of age.
Complications	N/A
Associated Diseases	◘ **Guillain–Barré Syndrome** An acute inflammatory demyelinating polyradiculoneuropathy usually triggered by viral (CMV, EBV) or bacterial (*Campylobacter jejuni* gastroenteritis) infection; presents with bilaterally symmetrical, areflexic, ascending motor weakness; associated with paresthesias and autonomic disturbances; LP shows increased CSF protein without cellular infiltrate (cyto-albuminic dissociation); treat with

plasmapheresis or intravenous immunoglobulins; intubate if complicated by respiratory muscle paralysis.

ID/CC	An 8-year-old male presents with **fever** and chills for three days associated with **fatigue, joint pain,** sore throat, and an **extensive skin rash on his left leg.**
HPI	The patient is a native of **Wisconsin** who attended a **summer camp** seven days ago (incubation 3–30 days). On directed questioning, he recalls having noticed a **tick bite** on his leg while hiking in the forest.
PE	VS: normal. PE: neurologic exam normal; rash is **nonpruritic,** started as a red spot (erythematous macule) at site of tick bite, and continued to expand in a **ringlike manner with an active border and central clearing,** yielding a **target appearance** (= ERYTHEMA CHRONICUM MIGRANS).
Labs	CBC: no anemia or leukocytosis. Elevated ESR; **elevated IgM** for *Borrelia burgdorferi* initially (window period of two weeks); **elevated IgG** later (six weeks); false positives in other spirochete infections, collagen vascular diseases, leptospirosis, and mononucleosis; diagnosis **confirmed by Western blot;** positive blood culture. LP: lymphocytosis; mildly elevated protein; normal glucose.
Imaging	N/A
Pathogenesis	Caused by *Borrelia burgdorferi* (a spirochete), which is transmitted by the tick *Ixodes dammini.* Lyme disease initially presents with a diagnostic rash > 5 cm surrounding the area of the tick bite whose center may desquamate, ulcerate, or necrose, together with satellite lesions. **Stage I** is characterized by **erythema chronicum migrans,** severe headache, fever, chills, and malaise (atypical cases may resolve spontaneously). **Stage II** occurs weeks afterward and presents with **CNS symptoms** (transverse myelitis, meningoencephalitis, mononeuritis multiplex, dysesthesias, CN palsy, chorea) and **cardiac abnormalities** (conduction disturbances, myocarditis, arrhythmias). **Stage III** occurs months to years after initial infection and presents as recurrent, **migratory arthritis and synovitis** (silver stain for spirochetes positive, synovial fluid *Borrelia* DNA positive by PCR) and atrophic macules on the fingers and toes (= ACRODERMATITIS CHRONICA ATROPHICANS). Associated with HLA-DR4 (stage III).

Epidemiology	The **most common vector-borne disease** in the U.S., its incidence is increasing; found in the coastal Northeast, California, and the Midwest (clustered around woodlands). It is more common in the summer and early fall. The **tick bite** is usually painless (24-hour tick attachment is needed for transmission). Reservoir includes deer, mice, and raccoons.
Management	Pediatric disease can be managed with **amoxicillin** (avoid tetracycline). Prevention consists of avoidance, clothing protection and repellent, and appropriate, prompt tick removal. Consider post-tick-bite antibiotic prophylaxis if endemic. A vaccine is now available.
Complications	Dissemination (latent period lasts weeks to years), subacute encephalopathy, leukoencephalitis, cardiac conduction defects, and musculoskeletal disorders.
Associated Diseases	◻ **Acute Rheumatic Fever** A dysfunctional immune response to oropharyngeal infection with beta-hemolytic group A streptococcus leading to autoimmune tissue damage at characteristic body sites (especially joints, cardiac valves, and skin); presents 1–3 weeks after throat infection with migratory polyarthritis, endocarditis, subcutaneous nodules, and a peculiar skin rash (erythema marginatum); Sydenham's chorea may present as a late manifestation; ASO antibody titer elevated; culture of throat swab yields beta-hemolytic streptococcus; treat with high-dose aspirin, corticosteroids, prophylaxis of recurrences with monthly intramuscular benzathine penicillin; complications include CHF and permanent valvular disease.

◻ **Ehrlichiosis** Infection by tick-borne bacteria of *Ehrlichia* spp.; presents with fever, malaise, myalgia, headache, nausea, and vomiting; can cause severe pulmonary and CNS disease; leukopenia and thrombocytopenia; serologic confirmation by elevated antibody titer on indirect immunofluorescence; treat with doxycycline; complications include seizures and coma.

◻ **Juvenile Rheumatoid Arthritis** Arthritis striking before age 16; presents with fever, skin rash, and tender swelling of the knee joints (the most common joints |

affected); normochromic, normocytic anemia, elevated ESR, and rheumatoid factor negative; synovial fluid shows leukocytosis; treat with NSAIDs, intra-articular corticosteroids for refractory disease; complications include iridocyclitis, which can lead to blindness.

◪ **Rocky Mountain Spotted Fever** Caused by *Rickettsia rickettsii;* vector is wood tick; presents with a peripheral petechial rash on the palms and soles; positive Weil–Felix reaction; treat with chloramphenicol and tetracyclines.

ID/CC	A **16-month-old** girl presents to the emergency room with failure to thrive, fever, cough, and a **rash of one week's duration.**
HPI	Her parents report that the child has become increasingly irritable and fatigued and has demonstrated increasingly poor oral intake over the past week. They add that she has also had a persistent, nonproductive **cough,** a runny nose **(coryza),** sneezing, and **conjunctivitis.** Three days ago the parents noted a red **rash that appeared first on the face** and behind the ears and then **"moved" down to the trunk and palms.** The child's fever was as high as 40 C but is now decreasing.
PE	VS: fever (39.1 C); tachycardia (HR 130); tachypnea (RR 24). PE: small, poorly nourished, and in moderate distress; erythematous, nonpruritic, **maculopapular rash** noted along length of trunk and bilateral palms and soles with some confluence of lesions; mild brownish discoloration of skin; small, 1- to 2-mm **bluish-white spots** (= KOPLIK'S SPOTS) noted on inflamed, erythematous oral mucous membranes and buccal mucosa; mild **oropharyngeal edema** with yellow exudate on tonsils; moderate cervical lymphadenopathy bilaterally; lungs clear.
Labs	CBC: WBC count 1,800. UA: 2+ protein on urine dipstick.
Imaging	CXR: normal (may often be abnormal owing to frequent secondary bacterial pneumonias).
Pathogenesis	The measles virus invades the respiratory epithelium and spreads via blood to the skin, respiratory tract, GI tract, and reticuloendothelial system, where it infects all WBC types. Virions are generally transmitted by respiratory secretions, predominantly through aerosol exposure but also through direct contact; patients are contagious 1–2 days before the onset of symptoms until four days after the rash appears. The mean interval from infection to onset of symptoms is approximately 10 days; the time to onset of rash is approximately 14 days.
Epidemiology	Measles has a worldwide distribution, and humans are the only natural hosts. A recent resurgence of cases has been noted during the 1990s due to failure to immunize infants and young children in the inner cities. However,

MEASLES

the standard vaccination protocol has resulted in the reporting of < 300 cases per year to the CDC. The majority of cases continue to be found in preschool children, with the highest mortality found in children < 2 years and among adults. Worldwide pediatric mortality continues to be > 1 million each year.

Management

Primary prevention is central to disease control. The current recommendation suggests that the first **vaccination** be given between the ages of 12 and 15 months and the second at 4–6 years (prior to entry into school). Preschool children < 1 year may be given their initial vaccination as early as six months in the presence of outbreaks. Susceptible individuals exposed to the measles virus can be treated with live virus vaccine to prevent disease if given within five days of exposure; this should be followed with gamma globulin within days of the exposure and by live measles vaccine three months later. The vaccine should not be used in pregnant women or immune-compromised individuals. Patients with measles should be **isolated** for one week following the development of the rash.

Complications

The mortality rate of this condition is 0.6%; death is primarily related to CNS encephalitis and bacterial pneumonias. Respiratory complications include viral bronchopneumonia or bronchiolitis (1%–7%); CNS complications are common and include acute encephalitis (fever, headache, drowsiness, coma, and seizures), which occurs in 1 in 1,000 patients, has an onset 3–7 days after the rash, and carries a high mortality rate (10%–20%). **Subacute sclerosing panencephalitis** is an extremely rare complication (1 in 100,000) involving a delayed neurodegenerative process; usually seen following infection in males < 2 years old, this entity manifests as progressive dementia years after the initial infection. Secondary bacterial infections such as otitis media (the most frequent complication) and cervical adenitis are common; GI complications such as gastroenteritis, hepatitis, appendicitis, ileocolitis, and mesenteric adenitis are also seen.

Associated Diseases

N/A

ID/CC	A 1-month-old male infant presents with **marked muscle rigidity and spasm.**
HPI	The mother did not receive any prenatal care, and the child was delivered at home. The child has **not received any immunizations.**
PE	VS: tachycardia; tachypnea. PE: extremely ill-looking with **generalized rigidity** and **opisthotonos; spasm worsens** with agitation; jaw muscle rigidity (= TRISMUS).
Labs	CBC/Lytes/ABGs: normal. Culture of **umbilical stump** yields *Clostridium tetani.*
Imaging	N/A
Pathogenesis	Caused by *Clostridium tetani,* a **gram-positive, motile, nonencapsulated, anaerobic, spore-bearing bacillus** that produces a **powerful neurotoxin** (tetanospasmin). The toxin acts principally on **the spinal cord** (inhibits the release of glycine, an inhibitory neurotransmitter). The characteristic clinical features are determined by the relative strengths of the opposing muscles. For example, the greater strength of the masseter over the opposing digastricus and mylohyoid results in **trismus.** The combination of flexion of the upper extremities and extension of the lower extremities is termed **opisthotonos.**
Epidemiology	The cause of numerous infant deaths in developing countries, most attributable to the lack of tetanus immunization and the use of contaminated material to cut the umbilical cord.
Management	Provide ventilatory assistance; maintain nutrition and fluid and electrolyte balance; give **IM tetanus IgG.** Give **penicillin G;** control tetanic spasms with diazepam/phenobarbital. **Debride devitalized tissue** where *C. tetani* is growing. **Immunize pregnant women** with tetanus toxoid and maintain proper asepsis during delivery.
Complications	Notable complications include aspiration pneumonia, **respiratory failure,** rhabdomyolysis (from sustained seizure activity), and autonomic nervous system dysfunction (cardiac arrhythmias, unstable BP, temperature instability, and epileptic seizures).

NEONATAL TETANUS

ID/CC	A 10-month-old infant presents with complaints of **severe, intractable, chronic diarrhea** and **failure to thrive.**
HPI	The father reveals that the **mother died of AIDS** shortly after delivery.
PE	VS: mild fever; tachycardia; tachypnea. PE: emaciated and grossly malnourished; oral **thrush;** axillary, cervical, and inguinal **lymphadenopathy; hepatosplenomegaly.**
Labs	**CD4 T-cell count depressed; ELISA** and **Western blot** for HIV-1 **positive** (could be due to maternal antibodies but strongly supports the diagnosis in the presence of symptoms); **PCR viral RNA positive** (confirming HIV infection).
Imaging	CXR: normal.
Pathogenesis	Transmission of HIV-1 from mother to infant most commonly occurs **during delivery** through contact with contaminated blood or secretions. **Transplacental** passage of the virus and postnatal infection through **breast feeding** also occur. Increased risk of infection in the neonate is associated with advanced disease in the mother (**p24 antigenemia,** high level of **HIV-1 RNA** in plasma, and **low CD4+** cell counts).
Epidemiology	Transmission of HIV-1 from mother to infant varies from 13% to 45% in cohort studies conducted in Europe and Africa, respectively, with an average of approximately 25%.
Management	**Zidovudine (AZT)** administered during the **second** and **third trimesters, intrapartum,** and during **the first six weeks of life** reduces transmission. Antiretroviral therapy is started when immune suppression or HIV-related symptoms are demonstrated. Administer *Pneumocystis carinii* pneumonia prophylaxis and antimicrobials for specific infections. Pregnancy should be discouraged in female carriers. Children with AIDS should not be given oral polio vaccine, BCG, or MMR. DTP, hepatitis B, and inactivated polio vaccine can be administered. HIV-positive mothers **should not breast feed** their babies.
Complications	N/A

Associated Diseases

◘ **HIV Transmission in Pregnancy** Vertical transmission of HIV most commonly occurring in the third trimester or during birth; presents with acute retroviral syndrome (e.g., fever, malaise, adenopathy) in the first months of life; PCR detection of HIV from newborn's blood; prevention is the treatment; give AZT to the mother during the third trimester or at least during labor, markedly diminishing the rate of transmission (from 24% to 8%).

ID/CC	A 7-year-old boy presents with **fever, pain and swelling of the elbows and knees,** and a **skin rash** on his trunk and arms of two days' duration.
HPI	The patient is otherwise healthy with no relevant past medical history. Two weeks ago, he suffered from a **sore throat,** high **fever,** and generalized weakness. He has no history of tick bites.
PE	VS: **fever** (38.5 C); tachycardia; normal BP. PE: **confluent, serpiginous, nonpruritic erythematous rash** over trunk and proximal extremities (= ERYTHEMA MARGINATUM); **subcutaneous nodules** (which are painless, firm, and 3–4 mm in diameter) on extensor tendons of MCP joints and elbow as well as on posterior scalp; swollen, red knee and elbow joints (= POLYARTHRITIS); pedal edema; elevated JVP; high-frequency apical systolic murmur with radiation to axilla (mitral insufficiency due to carditis); bilateral fine inspiratory rales; mild tender hepatomegaly.
Labs	CBC: **leukocytosis** (14,900) with **neutrophilia** (85%). **Increased ASO** titer and anti-DNase (evidence of preceding streptococcal infection); **elevated ESR** (useful for following disease activity; remains elevated for months); elevated C-reactive protein (CRP); culture of throat swab grows *Streptococcus pyogenes*; blood culture negative. ECG: changing P-wave contour and **prolonged PR interval with small QRS complexes** (due to ventricular dilatation and small pericardial effusion).
Imaging	CXR: **cardiomegaly;** increased pulmonary vascular markings; very small left pleural effusion. Echo: vegetations over the mitral valve with regurgitation.
Pathogenesis	A sequela of infection with **group A beta-hemolytic streptococci** that causes autoimmune heart damage; it typically occurs two weeks after streptococcal pharyngitis (unlike glomerulonephritis, carditis does not follow skin infections). **Jones' major criteria** for the diagnosis of rheumatic fever include **pancarditis** (clinical or radiologic evidence of myocarditis, endocarditis, and pericarditis), **polyarthritis** (typically migratory arthritis involving large joints), **Sydenham's chorea** (more frequent in females; involuntary purposeful movements of voluntary muscles), **subcutaneous nodules,** and

erythema marginatum (migratory pink macular rash seen on the trunk and proximal extremities). **Minor criteria** include **fever, arthralgia, previous rheumatic fever, elevated ESR, elevated CRP,** and **prolonged PR interval.** The presence of **two major or one major and two minor** criteria plus evidence of a **recent strep infection** (elevated ASO titers, positive throat culture for *S. pyogenes*) is used to diagnose acute rheumatic fever.

Epidemiology	The leading cause of acquired heart disease in children, it usually occurs between the ages of 5 and 15.
Management	Treat infection. Give aspirin, steroids, bed rest. Administer digoxin and diuretics in the presence of CHF and phenobarbital or diazepam for chorea. ESR takes months to return to normal. Prophylaxis every month with benzathine penicillin to prevent recurrences (more common in younger children and in those who had carditis; usually appears in the first few years post-rheumatic fever).
Complications	Arrhythmias, pericardial effusion, pneumonitis, and valvular heart defects (more commonly affects the mitral valve).
Associated Diseases	◘ **Henoch–Schönlein Purpura** A self-limiting purpuric vasculitis due to immune complex deposition; common in children; presents with a palpable puerperal rash on the buttocks and legs, abdominal pain, fever, and arthralgia; renal biopsy reveals segmental glomerulonephritis with crescents and mesangial IgA deposition; treatment is not required; complications include very rare progression to glomerulonephritis.
	◘ **Juvenile Rheumatoid Arthritis** Arthritis striking before age 16; presents with fever, skin rash, and tender swelling of the knee joints (the most common joints affected); normochromic, normocytic anemia, elevated ESR, and rheumatoid factor negative; synovial fluid shows leukocytosis; treat with NSAIDs, intra-articular corticosteroids for refractory disease; complications include iridocyclitis, which can lead to blindness.
	◘ **Lyme Disease** Caused by the spirochete *Borrelia burgdorferi;* the vector is the *Ixodes* tick; presents with a

migrating, target-shaped, erythematous rash called erythema migrans as well as with lymphadenopathy and arthritis; positive IgM ELISA for *B. burgdorferi;* treat with doxycycline.

ID/CC	A 9-year-old Boy Scout presents with **sudden-onset fever, chills, headache, lethargy,** and **abdominal pain** of four days' duration.
HPI	Earlier today he developed a **rash that began on his wrists and ankles** and spread to the trunk. He is a healthy boy with no relevant past medical history who went **camping in North Carolina** 10 days ago. Directed questioning reveals that he suffered a **tick bite** on his lower leg.
PE	VS: **fever** (39.1 C); tachycardia (HR 129); normal BP. PE: slight **icterus;** face flushed and **conjunctiva injected;** generalized nontender rash of small, bright red confluent macules (early) and petechiae (later), some of them hemorrhagic and necrotic, on soles, palms, wrists, ankles, arms, trunk, and abdomen (due to vasculitis); mild hepatosplenomegaly.
Labs	CBC: slight **leukopenia** (5,000); thrombocytopenia. Lytes: hyponatremia. UA: proteinuria. Skin biopsy (positive early) and serologic immunofluorescence positive for *Rickettsia rickettsii;* Weil–Felix positive.
Imaging	N/A
Pathogenesis	Caused by *Rickettsia rickettsii* and transmitted by *Dermacentor andersoni* tick bite; characterized by a **typical triad** of **history of tick exposure, fever,** and **generalized centripetal rash.** The rash **characteristically involves the palms and soles.** At times, however, the disease appears without a rash.
Epidemiology	Commonly occurs in the spring and summer; the incubation period is usually 2–14 days. More prevalent on the **East Coast** (primarily in Virginia and North Carolina) and in Oklahoma. The overall mortality rate is significantly reduced with treatment.
Management	Treat dehydration and electrolyte imbalance. Give **chloramphenicol** for at least one week for children < 8 years. **Doxycycline** may be given to older children.
Complications	Myocarditis, pneumonitis, gangrene of digits, acute renal failure, residual convulsions, DIC, and ARDS.
Associated Diseases	◼ **Lyme Disease** Caused by the spirochete *Borrelia burgdorferi;* the vector is the *Ixodes* tick; presents with a

migrating, target-shaped, erythematous rash called erythema migrans as well as with lymphadenopathy and arthritis; positive IgM ELISA for *B. burgdorferi;* treat with doxycycline.

◘ Disseminated Intravascular Coagulation A consumptive coagulopathy characterized by excessive thrombin activity that results in fibrin deposition with thrombus formation in the microcirculation; caused by septicemia, burns, trauma, metastatic malignancy, or obstetric complications; presents with profuse bleeding (with fresh frozen plasma, platelet transfusions, cryoprecipitate, fibrinogen, or thrombotic complications); schistocytes on peripheral blood smear; low fibrinogen and platelets, prolonged PT, and elevated fibrin split products; treat the underlying cause; treat bleeding complications (with fresh frozen plasma, platelets, cryoprecipitate, fibrinogen)

ID/CC	An 8-year-old female presents with **fever** of five days' duration and an **itchy skin rash** that **started on her face and trunk** and **spread to her extremities.**
HPI	Lesions have appeared in **successive crops.** Four classmates recently missed school due to similar symptoms.
PE	VS: **fever** (39.1 C); tachycardia. PE: well hydrated and nourished; lesions consist of **macules** (earliest), **papules, vesicles, pustules, and scabs, all present simultaneously** and appearing predominantly over trunk, face, and scalp; lungs clear; no hepatosplenomegaly; neurologic exam normal.
Labs	CBC: **leukopenia** (4,500). **Multinucleated giant cells** on Tzanck smears of vesicle base scraping; specific complement fixation and fluorescent antibody test positive.
Imaging	CXR: no evidence of pneumonitis (a potential complication).
Pathogenesis	Also known as **chickenpox;** caused by the **varicella-zoster virus** (a DNA herpesvirus). Spread by **direct contact** and **respiratory droplets.** Transmissible until lesions have crusted over.
Epidemiology	A **highly contagious** infection that occurs in epidemics; more common in **late winter** and **early spring.**
Management	Treat with **oral antihistamines** (avoid topical), **acetaminophen** (avoid aspirin due to risk of Reye's syndrome), oatmeal soap, and calamine lotion; clip fingernails (to prevent excoriation). Give prophylactic, postexposure **varicella-zoster immune globulin** to newborns, immune-compromised patients, pregnant mothers, and adults > 25 years old. **Acyclovir** can be given to immune-compromised patients and infants as well as in severe cases. Prevent through use of live attenuated vaccine.
Complications	Complications include **skin infection** (most common); myocarditis, thrombocytopenia (skin, mucous membranes and vesicle hemorrhages), scarlet fever (strep infection), encephalitis (varicella cerebellitis), **pneumonitis** (in older patients, carries risk of ARDS), **Reye's syndrome** (with ASA), **herpes zoster** (=

SHINGLES; reactivation of dormant virus in nerves), and visceral involvement in immune-compromised patients (transplant patients, cancer patients undergoing chemotherapy, those on steroids, patients with HIV). In pregnant patients, complications can include low weight, deafness, cataracts, and chorioretinitis in the fetus.

Associated Diseases ◘ **Reye's Syndrome** An idiopathic disorder linked to children with influenza B and varicella infection who have been treated with salicylates; presents with coma, fever, and hepatomegaly; impaired liver function; CT shows cerebral edema; treat with emergent liver transplantation.

ID/CC	A 2-year-old **boy** presents with fever, cough, and irritability.
HPI	He contracted his first respiratory tract infection at approximately nine months of age and has had numerous **bacterial infections** since then.
PE	VS: fever (39 C); tachypnea (RR 40); tachycardia (HR 130). PE: grunting respirations; **tonsils absent on inspection;** flaring of alae nasi; intercostal retractions; use of accessory muscles of respiration; **crackles at right base** (pneumonia).
Labs	CBC: elevated WBC (15,000); normal lymphocyte counts. Sputum Gram stain reveals gram-positive cocci in chains; **markedly depressed IgA, IgG, and IgM levels; total immunoglobulin levels < 100 mg/dL; lymph node biopsy reveals absence of germinal centers.**
Imaging	CXR: focal right lower lobe infiltrate.
Pathogenesis	Also known as **X-linked agammaglobulinemia;** caused by a **defect in a nonreceptor tyrosine kinase** involved in signal transduction; the defect leads to a developmental block and arrest at the pre-B-cell level. A small number of B cells progress to maturation and exist in the periphery as plasma cells; however, this occurs at a relatively low frequency. As a result, patients are **highly susceptible to bacterial infections,** particularly within the respiratory tract and by encapsulated organisms.
Epidemiology	Develops in **boys,** with the first sequelae of the disease appearing late in the first year of life following the disappearance of maternal immunoglobulins. Females may serve as carriers but are unaffected.
Management	Administer **monthly IV immunoglobulin,** which replenishes IgG but not IgA. Doses should be titrated to maintain a trough IgG level in excess of 400 mg/dL.
Complications	Patients may develop chronic meningoencephalitis secondary to echovirus infection, dermatomyositis, arthritis similar to rheumatoid arthritis, and diarrhea secondary to *Giardia lamblia.*
Associated Diseases	N/A

ID/CC	An 8-month-old male is seen for **gradual-onset breathing difficulties** (due to *Pneumocystis carinii* pneumonia).
HPI	The child also has a low-grade **fever,** a nonproductive **cough,** and **chronic diarrhea.** His mother states that he also has a history of **multiple candidal skin infections.**
PE	VS: **fever; tachypnea;** tachycardia; normal BP. PE: **cachectic;** cyanosis and dyspnea noted; **alopecia** (almost universal feature) with abundant **seborrhea** on scalp and forehead; scattered rales in lungs.
Labs	CBC: **marked lymphopenia;** neutropenia; **anemia** (of chronic disease); increased platelets (= THROMBOCYTOSIS). Anergic response to PPD; hypogammaglobulinemia; increased lymphocyte AMP; **low adenosine deaminase** (ADA) **activity in RBCs.** ABGs: hypoxemia.
Imaging	CXR: **no thymic shadow** (= THYMIC APLASIA). **[A]** CXR: patchy infiltrates bilaterally (atypical pneumonia).
Pathogenesis	Severe combined immunodeficiency is a heterogeneous group of disorders caused by **defective lymphocyte development.** Defective B-lymphocyte development results in **humoral immune deficiency (hypogammaglobulinemia);** defective T-lymphocyte development results in **cellular immune deficiency** (absent delayed-type hypersensitivity). **ADA deficiency** is a variant that accounts for 20% of cases. Most patients present with *Pneumocystis* pneumonia.
Epidemiology	A relatively rare immune deficiency; most patients die within the first year of life due to sepsis.
Management	**Bone marrow transplant** offers the best chance of cure. Start TMP-SMX for *Pneumocystis* **prophylaxis; IgG replacement** when the diagnosis is known. Give antibiotics for infection; avoid blood transfusions (graft-versus-host disease).
Complications	N/A
Associated Diseases	◻ **Chédiak–Higashi Syndrome** An autosomal-recessive defect of microtubule polymerization leading to impaired chemotaxis and phagocytosis; presents with

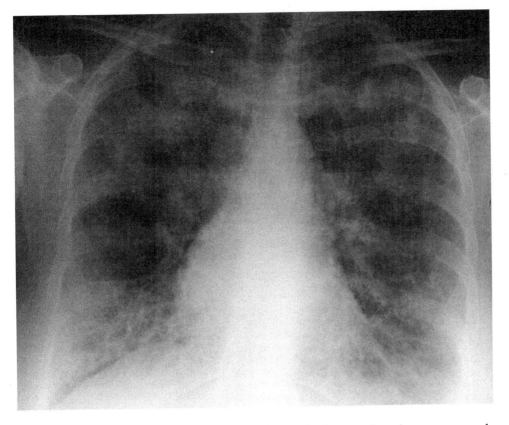

recurrent pyogenic staphylococcal and streptococcal infections; decreased neutrophil count and large cytoplasmic granules; treat with antibiotics appropriate to infection.

◘ **Chronic Granulomatous Disease** An X-linked disorder due to a deficiency of NADPH oxidase; presents with recurrent staphylococcal and fungal infections; neutrophilic leukocytosis and absence of respiratory burst; treat infections appropriately; consider chronic Bactrim prophylaxis.

◘ **Wiskott–Aldrich Syndrome** An X-linked recessive disease; presents with epistaxis, eczema, and recurrent infections; thrombocytopenia and inability to form antibody to carbohydrate antigen; reduced IgM levels; treat by bone marrow transplantation; patients are at increased risk of developing lymphomas.

ID/CC	A newborn infant with a **low Apgar** score is evaluated.
HPI	The neonate has been **cyanotic since birth,** and his color does not improve when he cries (unlike choanal atresia). The mother did not undergo any prenatal ultrasound screening for birth defects.
PE	Full-term male neonate with cyanosis; **breath sounds absent on left side; heart sounds shifted** toward right; occasional **peristaltic movements heard over left side of chest;** abdomen is scaphoid.
Labs	ABGs: hypoxemia.
Imaging	CXR: **loops of intestine herniating through the diaphragmatic defect** into the left side of the chest with the heart shifted toward the right. [A] CXR: another case demonstrates a right diaphragmatic defect and bowel loops in the right thorax (1), displacing the esophagus (NG tube) (2) to the left. US-Fetal: bowel loops in chest with incomplete diaphragm.
Pathogenesis	There are two types of congenital diaphragmatic hernia; most commonly, a posterolateral defect in the diaphragm **(Bochdalek hernia)** is involved, but approximately 5% of cases are due to a retrosternal defect **(Morgagni hernia).** These defects allow abdominal viscera to enter the thorax and compromise lung development. Embryologically, the diaphragm is derived from the septum transversum, pleuroperitoneal folds, dorsal esophageal mesentery, and body wall.
Epidemiology	**Ninety percent** of diaphragmatic hernias occur on the **left side.**
Management	**Ventilatory support** and **surgical repair** are required. Restrictive lung disease, reactive lung disease, neurologic abnormalities, pectus excavatum, scoliosis, and recurrent herniation may result. High-frequency ventilation or extracorporeal membrane oxygenation (ECMO) may be needed to treat pulmonary hypertension.
Complications	Pulmonary hypertension due to prolonged intubation; infections.
Associated Diseases	N/A

CONGENITAL DIAPHRAGMATIC HERNIA

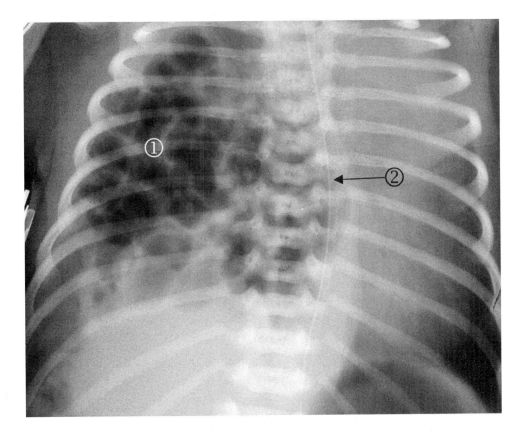

CONGENITAL DIAPHRAGMATIC
HERNIA

ID/CC	A **1-day-old** male is seen by a neonatologist for **failure to pass meconium** and persistent **bilious vomiting** after each feeding.
HPI	The infant is the first-born child of a healthy 40-year-old woman who had **polyhydramnios.** The child was born **premature** at 32 weeks' gestation and suffers from **Down's syndrome.**
PE	VS: normal. PE: **hypotonic** and mildly dehydrated with dry mucous membranes; flattened face, low-set ears, macroglossia, flattened nasal bridge, and **epicanthal folds** (all consistent with Down's syndrome); **abdomen distended** and tympanic to percussion; **visible peristalsis.**
Labs	CBC: normal. Lytes: hypokalemia; hyponatremia; hypochloremia. BUN slightly increased with normal creatinine (dehydration). ABGs: metabolic alkalosis (vomiting, loss of hydrochloric acid). Karyotype: trisomy 21.
Imaging	**[A]** XR-Abdomen: dilatation of the gastric chamber (1) and proximal duodenum (2) with no air in the remainder of the bowel, producing the typical image ("double bubble"). **[B]** US-Fetal: another case with dilated fluid-filled stomach (1) and duodenum (2). BE: normal (rule out malrotation).
Pathogenesis	Duodenal atresia occurs as a result of failure of the second part of the duodenum to canalize during embryonic development. It is commonly associated with prematurity, **polyhydramnios,** and **Down's syndrome** and typically presents with **bilious vomiting** during the **first day of life.**
Epidemiology	After the ileum, the duodenum is the most common site of congenital intestinal atresia.
Management	**Restoration of fluid and electrolyte balance** is of paramount importance. **Nasogastric suction** is instituted to decompress the abdomen and relieve signs of obstruction (> 40 cc of residual gastric material is diagnostic of obstruction), followed by **surgical repair.** Treatment usually involves a side-to-side duodeno-duodenostomy with a protective tube gastrostomy.

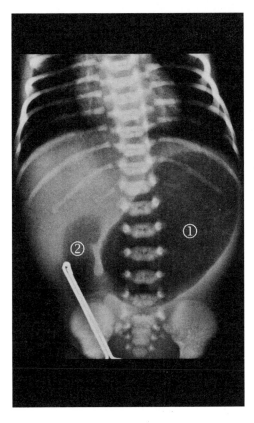

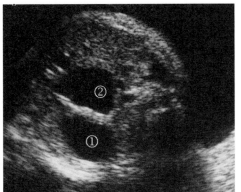

Complications	N/A
Associated Diseases	◘ **Hirschsprung's Disease** Congenital absence of parasympathetic myenteric ganglion cells in the rectum and sigmoid colon; shows a familial tendency and is more common in males; presents with abdominal distention and failure to pass stools in young children, rectal exam reveals an empty contracted rectum; baby passes stools following the rectal exam; XR of abdomen shows dilated colon proximal to the obstructing aganglionic segment; rectal biopsy (pathognomonic) reveals aganglionosis; treat by surgical excision of denervated bowel (narrowed segment).

◘ **Meconium Ileus** Intestinal obstruction in the neonatal period due to accumulation of viscous, inspissated meconium; commonly seen in cystic fibrosis; presents with abdominal distention and failure to pass meconium after birth; treat with Gastrografin enema, surgical laparotomy if refractory.

ID/CC	A **1-day-old** male presents with **yellowing of the skin and eyes** and **generalized swelling of the body** (= ANASARCA).
HPI	The **amniotic fluid** was **yellow** and the **placenta was enlarged** at the time of delivery. The child's mother is an otherwise-healthy 24-year-old **white** female who is **Rh negative.** This is her **second child.**
PE	VS: tachycardia. PE: generalized edema; marked **jaundice** with **yellow vernix; petechiae** on legs and arms; muscular **hypotonia** and **lethargy** (severe disease); decreased breath sounds in left lung field (due to pleural effusion); abdominal exam reveals **hepatosplenomegaly** (compensatory extramedullary erythropoiesis) and ascites.
Labs	CBC/PBS: **anemia** (7 mg/dL); thrombocytopenia; polychromasia; **nucleated erythrocytes** (= ERYTHROBLASTS); **direct Coombs' test positive** (child's serum); **indirect Coombs' test positive** (antibodies in maternal blood); anti-Rh agglutinins positive in infant's blood. LFTs: **increased indirect bilirubin** (due to hemolysis).
Imaging	CXR: mild left pleural effusion. KUB: ascites.
Pathogenesis	Erythroblastosis fetalis can occur in **Rh-positive fetuses** of previously **sensitized Rh-negative mothers.** During the first pregnancy, Rh-positive fetal erythrocytes reach the maternal circulation (in the third trimester and during delivery) and stimulate antibody production against the Rh antigen. In subsequent pregnancies, these maternal antibodies pass to the fetus via the placenta and destroy fetal erythrocytes (if Rh positive). This hemolysis leads to compensatory overproduction of nucleated erythrocytes (= ERYTHROBLASTS). The clinical spectrum of disease ranges from mild anemia and jaundice to erythroblastosis fetalis to hydrops fetalis. ABO incompatibility rarely leads to erythroblastosis fetalis.
Epidemiology	More common in **whites. Predisposing factors** include prematurity, C-section, abortion, breech, short interval between pregnancies, eclampsia, and amniocentesis.
Management	Treat with **phenobarbital** (reduces bilirubin) prior to

delivery. If the mother's Rh Ab titer > 1:32, perform paired amniocentesis. If titers rise, do intrauterine transfusion. **Induce labor** in the presence of previous severe hemolytic disease or if hydrops is seen on ultrasound. Perform **exchange transfusion** in the presence of jaundice at birth, kernicterus, bilirubin > 15 mg/dL, a rise in indirect bilirubin > 0.5 mg/dL/hr or cord bilirubin > 4.0 mg/dL, methemalbuminemia, or anemia < 45 HT. Cross-match type O Rh-negative whole blood and exchange. **Phototherapy** may be used in ABO disease if bilirubin > 10 and may be used in Rh disease in conjunction with transfusion. Late anemia may occur after days or weeks and is more frequent in Rh than in ABO incompatibility. To prevent this complication, administer **RhoGAM** intramuscularly immediately after delivery for Rh-negative mothers (prevents sensitization). Also give for ectopic pregnancy and induced or spontaneous abortion.

Complications

Complications include stillbirths, hydrops fetalis, and **kernicterus** that may proceed to potentially fatal brain damage (bilirubin deposition in basal ganglia). The risk of kernicterus increases with hypoglycemia, drugs that displace bilirubin from albumin (sulfisoxazole), acidosis, hypoxia, hypothermia, and indirect bilirubin > 20 mg/dL. Sequelae include mental retardation, cerebral palsy, and sensorineural deafness.

Associated Diseases

◘ **Rh Incompatibility** Rh-negative mother produces anti-D antibodies to Rh-positive infant, producing hemolysis; presents with edema, jaundice, and cyanosis in newborn; positive direct Coombs' test and increased indirect bilirubin; treat with UV lamp therapy and exchange transfusion.

◘ **Thalassemia** An inherited defect of the alpha or beta chain of hemoglobin; common in African (beta defects), Southeast Asian (alpha defect), and Mediterranean populations; presents with chronic anemia of variable severity; seen on blood smear; increased fetal hemoglobin and increased HbA2 on electrophoresis; treat with blood transfusions, folic acid supplements, and iron chelation therapy due to risk of iron overload from chronic transfusion.

ID/CC	A 32-week-gestation (**premature**) male infant has bluish skin (= CYANOSIS) after delivery by cesarean section.
HPI	His mother had **third-trimester bleeding** and uterine contractions that did not stop with rest or medical management. The child's **Apgar score was low** at five minutes (6).
PE	VS: marked **tachypnea;** tachycardia; **hypothermia; hypotension.** PE: infant weighs 1.85 kg; uses **accessory muscles** of respiration; **nasal flaring; intercostal** and supraclavicular **retractions; cyanosis** of lips and fingers; **grunting; tubular breath sounds and rales.**
Labs	ABGs: **hypoxemia; hypercapnia;** mixed respiratory/metabolic (= LACTIC) acidosis. **Decreased lecithin-to-sphingomyelin (L/S) ratio in amniotic fluid.**
Imaging	**[A]** CXR: indistinct diaphragm; **reticular pulmonary infiltrates bilaterally** and diffuse **atelectasis** with increased lung field opacification and **air bronchograms** (signs may not be present in first 6–12 hours). **[B]** CXR: normal premature neonatal chest film for comparison.
Pathogenesis	Caused by a **deficiency of surfactant** (lipoprotein produced by type II pneumocytes, which decrease surface tension and stabilize alveoli) that results in atelectasis. **Atelectasis** and **decreased compliance** lead in turn to greatly increased effort to expand the lungs with subsequent respiratory failure, as well as to a very low functional residual capacity, hypoventilation, pulmonary vasoconstriction, **shunting, hypoxia, cyanosis,** and acidosis. Presents at birth or shortly thereafter.
Epidemiology	The most common cause of respiratory distress in **premature infants;** incidence is 5% at 35–36 weeks' gestational age (GA) and > 50% at 26–28 weeks' GA. Associated with **cesarean births, infants of diabetic mothers, fetal distress,** and **obstetrical bleeding.**
Management	Intubation, **ventilatory support; fluid, acid-base,** and **electrolyte balance; antibiotics** if infection is suspected. Give **betamethasone** to nondiabetic pregnant women to increase fetal lung maturity; **surfactant** in premature infants. Infants generally improve 3–7 days after onset.
Complications	Complications often stem from supportive care:

HYALINE MEMBRANE DISEASE

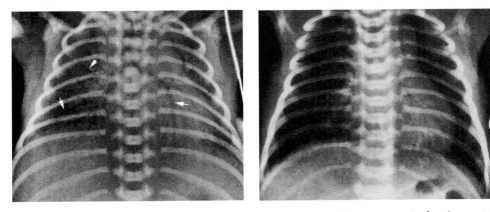

umbilical catheterization predisposes to infection and thrombosis; oxygen and pressure from ventilators may lead to **bronchopulmonary dysplasia; delayed closure of PDA** results from hypoxia, acidosis, and immaturity.

Associated Diseases
◻ **Meconium Aspiration** The most common cause of neonatal respiratory distress in full-term infants; due to bronchial obstruction by meconium; presents with acute cyanosis at birth; CXR shows consolidation and atelectasis and small pleural effusions; treat with aggressive suctioning, intubation if necessary, high-flow oxygen.

ID/CC	A **4-week-old male** infant is brought to the pediatrician because he has been **regurgitating** his food and has been having occasional bouts of vomiting for the past week.
HPI	The infant continues to have a **voracious appetite.** Earlier that day he presented with **nonbilious projectile vomiting** both during and immediately after feeding.
PE	VS: moderate tachycardia. PE: **lethargic** and mildly **dehydrated; low weight for age;** abdomen soft and flat; after nasogastric tube gastric emptying, 2-cm, firm, nontender, motile **olive-shaped mass** palpable in right upper quadrant; **peristalsis visible.**
Labs	CBC: increased hematocrit (hemoconcentration secondary to dehydration). Lytes: **hypokalemia; hyponatremia; hypochloremia.** ABGs: metabolic alkalosis (due to loss of hydrochloric acid). Elevated serum gastrin levels. ECG: flattened T wave; prominent U waves (hypokalemia).
Imaging	**[A]** UGI (with barium or water-soluble media): enlargement of the stomach chamber with increased peristalsis and delayed emptying with **string sign** (1) (narrowing and elongation of the pyloric canal). **[B]** US: **identification of hypertrophied muscle** (false negatives occur; pyloric muscle thickness > 4 mm).
Pathogenesis	Idiopathic. Longitudinal and circular muscle fibers in the distal stomach and pyloric region are hypertrophied. This results in gastric outlet obstruction, poor feeding, abdominal distention after feeding, and vomiting. The vomiting progresses in frequency and force, ultimately leading to projectile vomiting. Vomit may contain blood but generally does not contain bile (obstruction proximal to the ampulla of Vater).
Epidemiology	Relatively common cause of vomiting (1 in 500 births). More common in **male** and **full-term** infants. Higher risk in monozygotic twins. Onset of symptoms is usually in the **second or third week.**
Management	Perform **nasogastric tube** decompression; rehydrate and correct electrolyte imbalances. The definitive treatment is **Fredet–Ramstedt pyloromyotomy.**
Complications	Hypokalemic, hypochloremic metabolic alkalosis (tetany), reflux esophagitis, weight loss and starvation,

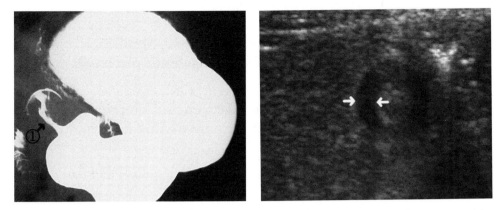

dehydration, unconjugated hyperbilirubinemia with jaundice (increased enterohepatic circulation), aspiration pneumonia, gastritis with bleeding (stasis), and learning disabilities if period of inanition was prolonged.

Associated Diseases

◘ **Intestinal Malrotation with Volvulus** Congenital failure of the colon to rotate properly during embryogenesis, allowing the small bowel to twist within the mesentery due to lack of proper peritoneal attachment; presents with bilious vomiting, abdominal distention, and fever; abdominal XR shows air-fluid levels and lack of gas in the colon; CT or barium enema reveals the cecum to lie outside the right lower quadrant; treatment is emergent laparotomy with reduction of volvulus.

◘ **Meckel's Diverticulum** The most common congenital anomaly of the GI tract; due to persistence of the vitelline duct or yolk sac; affects young children; presents with vomiting, hematochezia, distended abdomen, and a sausage-shaped mass in the right lower quadrant; anemia; nuclear imaging shows ectopic gastric mucosa; treat by surgical excision.

ID/CC	A **3-day-old** infant **delivered prematurely** develops **abdominal distention, lethargy, bilious vomiting, feeding intolerance,** and **bright red blood per rectum** (= HEMATOCHEZIA).
HPI	He is the first-born child of an apparently healthy mother who had presented with **amnionitis.** The child weighed 1.95 kg.
PE	VS: **hypothermia** with temperature instability; **bradycardia; hypotension.** PE: **lethargic** and icteric with periods of apnea; abdomen **distended and tympanic** with signs of **rigidity; absent bowel sounds;** marked rebound tenderness (peritonitis); **abdominal wall discoloration and "loopy" appearance.**
Labs	CBC: **polycythemia** (Hb 17.1); **marked leukocytosis** (may show neutropenia in severe septicemia); **thrombocytopenia.** Blood cultures yield *E. coli* and *Klebsiella*. ABGs: **metabolic acidosis.**
Imaging	**[A]** CXR: a different case demonstrating free subdiaphragmatic air (= PNEUMOPERITONEUM) (due to hollow viscus perforation). **[B]** KUB: edema of bowel wall; **pneumatosis intestinalis** (due to intramural gas); **intrahepatic portal venous gas** (late sign) and air-fluid levels may also be seen. BE is contraindicated (due to risk of perforation).
Pathogenesis	May be related to **ischemic insult** that damages the bowel lining and hampers mucus production, rendering the bowel susceptible to infection. Mucosal damage and colonization lead to intramural hemorrhage, mucosal edema, necrosis, ulceration, membrane formation, gangrene, and perforation. Associated with **prematurity,** polycythemia, congenital heart disease, umbilical catheterization, broad-spectrum antibiotics, and birth asphyxia. Affects the terminal ileum and right colon.
Epidemiology	A **common neonatal GI emergency.** Onset is usually on the third day of life. Mortality rate is approximately 30%.
Management	**Supportive management** (in ICU) addresses temperature, ventilation, circulation, and anemia; **x-ray every six hours** for the first 12–48 hours (high perforation risk); institute **GI rest** (NPO, GI suction,

NECROTIZING ENTEROCOLITIS

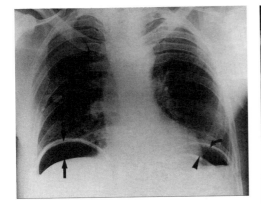

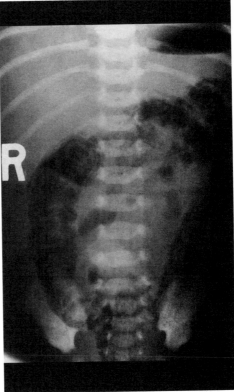

peripheral parenteral nutrition); maintain fluid and electrolyte balance. To **control infection,** give carbenicillin/gentamicin or clindamycin/aminoglycosides for gram-negative organisms (risk staphylococcal and *Candida* superinfection), vancomycin if clostridial. **Surgical resection** is required in the event of perforation, failure of medical therapy, abdominal wall cellulitis (erythema, warmth, induration), localized tenderness or mass > 12 hours, acidosis, or ascites.

Complications   **Strictures** may develop at the involved site; after resection, patients may develop **short bowel syndrome.**

Associated Diseases   N/A

ID/CC	A 2-week-old female presents with **lethargy**, yellowish eyes (= JAUNDICE), and **feeding difficulties.**
HPI	Her mother states that the infant sometimes has **fever** and at other times has a **low temperature** (temperature instability).
PE	VS: low-grade **fever** (38.1 C); tachycardia; tachypnea. PE: inconsolable with high-pitched cry; **bulging fontanelle;** during examination, patient has episode of **projectile vomiting.**
Labs	CBC: **leukocytosis with neutrophilia.** Lytes: normal. BUN and creatinine normal. LP: **increased pressure; neutrophilic pleocytosis; low glucose; increased protein.** Gram-positive cocci in chains seen on Gram stain; culture grows **group B streptococcus.**
Imaging	CT/MR-Brain: subtle meningeal thickening and enhancement.
Pathogenesis	The etiology of neonatal meningitis varies according to the time of onset. **Early-onset** infections (0–3 days) most frequently involve bacteremia with *E. coli* or *Streptococcus agalactiae* (= GROUP B STREP) and rarely lead to meningitis. **Late-onset** infections (14–28 days) are usually caused by **group B streptococcus** or *Listeria monocytogenes,* and **most progress** to meningitis. Early-onset infections are usually acquired perinatally from the maternal genital tract; late-onset infections are generally acquired from environmental (hospital or home) sources.
Epidemiology	N/A
Management	For neonatal meningitis, give **ampicillin** (covers *Listeria*) with **gentamicin** or with **cefotaxime.** For *Haemophilus* or *N. meningitides,* use ceftriaxone, cefuroxime, or ampicillin. For *S. pneumoniae,* treat with penicillin, ampicillin, or vancomycin. For TB, treat with INH and rifampin, streptomycin, and ethambutol. Corticosteroids are beneficial in *Haemophilus* meningitis.
Complications	Hydrocephalus, focal seizure, subdural effusion, brain abscess, and deafness. **FIRST AID 2** p. 202
Associated Diseases	◻ **Cryptococcal Meningitis** The most common fungal meningitis; may be acquired from inhalation of pigeon droppings; presents with headache, nuchal rigidity, and

cranial nerve palsies, usually in AIDS patients; LP shows elevated opening pressure, elevated protein, and decreased glucose; India ink reveals *Cryptococcus neoformans;* treat with amphotericin B.

◘ **Listeria Meningitis** Caused by *Listeria monocytogenes;* acquired in utero or through contaminated milk in neonates or in debilitated adults (e.g., alcoholics, immunosuppressed); presents with high fever, convulsions, and nuchal rigidity; neutrophilic leukocytosis; culture shows gram-positive bacillus; treat with IV ampicillin.

◘ **Meningococcemia** Systemically disseminated infection with *Neisseria meningitidis;* more commonly seen in those with terminal complement component (C5–C8) deficiency; presents with sudden fever, chills, severe headache, meningeal signs, and petechial rash; hypoglycemia, hyperkalemia, and hyponatremia; gram-negative diplococci in blood, possibly in CSF; gross pathology reveals bilateral adrenal hemorrhage; treat with penicillin G, rifampin for close contacts; complications include fulminant adrenal infarction; also called Waterhouse–Friderichsen syndrome.

ID/CC	A **5-day-old** female infant is seen for a **yellowish hue** in her eyes and skin (= JAUNDICE). The problem was **first noted on the third day of life** and has since worsened.
HPI	The infant is the **first-born** child of an apparently healthy white couple (G6PD unlikely). She is on formula food (no breast-milk jaundice). The mother denies any drug intake in the third trimester, and there is no family history of jaundice.
PE	VS: normal. PE: **well developed** and in **no acute distress; no cataracts** (vs. galactosemia); moderate **icterus** of conjunctiva, sublingual mucosa, and skin; **stool normal color; no hepatosplenomegaly** (vs. Rh incompatibility) and **no masses** (vs. choledochal cyst).
Labs	CBC/PBS: normal hemoglobin; normal erythrocyte morphology; hemoglobin electrophoresis normal; reticulocyte count normal. **Coombs' test negative.** LFTs: **indirect bilirubin markedly elevated** (9); **direct bilirubin mildly elevated** (1). Mother and infant Rh positive (no Rh incompatibility).
Imaging	N/A
Pathogenesis	Unconjugated bilirubin (major product of heme metabolism) is carried in the plasma by albumin and transported to the liver, where it is conjugated (by glucuronyl transferase) with glucuronic acid. Conjugated bilirubin is excreted with bile into the intestine, where the gut flora converts it to urobilinogen. Urobilinogen then returns to the liver via the enterohepatic circulation, is excreted in urine, or is converted to stercobilin and excreted in the feces. Neonates are predisposed to hyperbilirubinemia for various reasons, including (1) **increased bilirubin load** due to increased RBC mass and decreased RBC half-life; (2) **decreased** hepatic **glucuronyl transferase** activity; and (3) increased enterohepatic circulation and decreased conversion of bilirubin to urobilinogen (with subsequent reabsorption of bilirubin) because of decreased intestinal bacterial flora. Physiologic jaundice appears **after the first day,** peaks between the third and fifth day (more in prematures), and returns to normal in two weeks, with bilirubin that does not exceed 12 (15 in premature

PHYSIOLOGIC JAUNDICE OF NEWBORN

babies). The infant is otherwise normal. The diagnosis is one of exclusion.

Epidemiology	More common in Asians. Predisposing factors include **prematurity, dehydration,** and **malnutrition.**
Management	Usually **no treatment** is needed. **Phototherapy** or **exchange transfusion** may be used if bilirubin rises rapidly. Maintain good hydration and nutrition.
Complications	N/A
Associated Diseases	◘ **Thalassemia** An inherited defect of the alpha or beta chain of hemoglobin; common in African (beta defects), Southeast Asian (alpha defect), and Mediterranean populations; presents with chronic anemia of variable severity; target cells seen on blood smear; increased fetal hemoglobin and HbA2 on electrophoresis; treat with blood transfusions, folate supplements, and iron chelation therapy due to risk of iron overload from chronic transfusion.

◘ **Crigler–Najjar Syndrome** An inherited deficiency of glucuronyl transferase; presents with severe jaundice and kernicterus causing seizures in neonates; increased serum unconjugated bilirubin, and low fecal urobilinogen; treat with UV lamps and phenobarbital; complications include irreversible brain damage from kernicterus.

◘ **Gilbert's Syndrome** An autosomal-dominant, mild deficiency of glucuronyl transferase; presents with mild, episodic jaundice precipitated by stress; elevated unconjugated serum bilirubin; no treatment is required.

◘ **Hereditary Spherocytosis** An autosomal-dominant defect in erythrocyte cytoplasmic membrane structural proteins (e.g., spectrin), causing spherical erythrocytes; presents with chronic hemolytic anemia, jaundice, splenomegaly, and gallstones; anemia, spherocytes, reticulocytosis, osmotically fragile erythrocytes, and increased unconjugated serum bilirubin; splenectomy palliates symptoms and improves anemia; complications include aplastic crisis secondary to parvovirus B19 infection and cholecystitis.

PHYSIOLOGIC JAUNDICE OF NEWBORN

ID/CC	A **3-month-old** male infant cannot be awakened by his mother and has blue lips. When the paramedics arrive a few minutes later, it is clear that the child has been dead for at least four hours.
HPI	The infant was a **twin** and was the **second in order** of birth. Both parents are 19-year-old **Native Americans** who live in an **inner-city** area. The **mother smoked during pregnancy and did not receive prenatal care.** On directed questioning, the parents state that the child had had an **unusual cry** lately, together with episodes of **apnea, cyanosis,** and pallor. Last week he also had a **URI.**
PE	Autopsy showed petechiae on pericardial and pleural surfaces along with **gliosis of brainstem** and **hypertrophy of pulmonary smooth muscle** vasculature (long-existing hypoxia).
Labs	UA: toxicology screen negative.
Imaging	N/A
Pathogenesis	Sudden infant death syndrome (SIDS) is defined as an **unexplained sudden death** that cannot be accounted for by any abnormality on autopsy. Recurrent or chronic hypoxia may be caused by an abnormality in autonomic cardiopulmonary regulation.
Epidemiology	SIDS occurs in 1 in 350 live births and is the **most common cause of death in infants < 1 year of age.** It most commonly occurs during sleep, at night, and in infants aged **2–4 months** (rare before 1 month and after 9 months). Risk factors include poor and nonwhite infants, mothers who smoke or who have a history of substance abuse, prematurity, previous loss of an infant to SIDS, and URI.
Management	Provide **counseling** support for parents (for strong guilt feelings), continuing until and after parents decide to have a new baby. Impedance monitoring, performed at home for subsequent children as well as for children with apneic episodes, is warranted in some cases. Putting **infants to sleep on their back** decreases SIDS risk.
Complications	N/A
Associated Diseases	N/A

SUDDEN INFANT DEATH SYNDROME

ID/CC	A 5-year-old male presents with **malaise, periorbital edema, smoky-colored urine** (= HEMATURIA), abdominal pain with vomiting, and mild **fever**.
HPI	Ten days ago he had a **throat infection** (due to a nephritogenic strain of *Streptococcus*), from which he recovered uneventfully.
PE	VS: **hypertension** (BP 140/90). PE: mild **pallor;** no cyanosis or jaundice; **palpebral edema;** tonsils cryptic but no exudate; submaxillary glands palpable but nonpainful; regular rate and rhythm with no murmurs; no hepatosplenomegaly; **ankle edema** (2+); no skin rashes.
Labs	CBC: **anemia;** leukocytosis. **Increased ESR; increased BUN and creatinine.** ABGs: metabolic acidosis. Lytes: **hyperkalemia.** UA: **RBCs and RBC casts;** leukocyturia and proteinuria; hemoglobinuria. **C3 and total hemolytic complement** (CH_{50}) **low** (almost always); **increased ASO titer** (recent streptococcal infection); throat culture does not reveal *Streptococcus* (only 4% positive rate); ANA negative; DNase titer high.
Imaging	CXR/KUB: normal.
Pathogenesis	An immune complex disease that is usually caused by beta-hemolytic streptococcus types 12 and 49. Poststreptococcal glomerulonephritis occurs **10–14 days after strep infection.** Pathogenesis may be related to the deposition of streptococcal **antigen-antibody complexes in the glomeruli,** followed by activation of complement leading to inflammation. Electron microscopy reveals **electron-dense humps** (immune complexes) on the epithelial side of the glomerular basement membrane. Immunofluorescence demonstrates a granular pattern of immunoglobulin deposition.
Epidemiology	The most common childhood nephritis; affects preschool and school-age children. May be isolated or occur in epidemics. Occurs after tonsillitis, URIs, skin infection, and scarlet fever. A history of strep infection is found in 95% of cases.
Management	**Treat infection with penicillin** for 10 days to prevent spread of nephrogenic strain (erythromycin if allergic).

POSTSTREPTOCOCCAL GLOMERULONEPHRITIS

Diet high in carbohydrates and low in protein, sodium, potassium, and water. Treat **renal** and **cardiac failure** with peritoneal dialysis. Resolution may take 6–12 months (microscopic hematuria up to one year).

Complications

Cardiac failure, hypertensive encephalopathy (vomiting, severe headache, convulsions, visual disturbances), uremia, acute pulmonary edema, and chronic glomerulonephritis.

Associated Diseases

◘ **IgA Nephropathy** Also known as Berger's disease; idiopathic glomerulonephritis associated with upper respiratory or GI infections; presents with hematuria; elevated serum IgA; urine shows protein and red cell casts; renal biopsy shows IgA deposition; no effective treatment; almost half of all patients may progress to chronic renal failure.

◘ **Hemolytic-Uremic Syndrome** Acute renal failure and microangiopathic hemolytic anemia, usually associated with bacterial (*E. coli, Shigella*) infection in children or following cancer chemotherapy (mitomycin); presents with fever, malaise, hypotension, ecchymoses, periorbital edema, and oliguria; schistocytes seen on PBS; no evidence of DIC (normal PT, PTT, fibrinogen); thrombocytopenia and elevated BUN and creatinine; treat with plasmapheresis, IV fluids and pressors as needed to prevent acute renal failure and hemodynamic compromise.

◘ **Idiopathic Nephrotic Syndrome of Childhood** The most common cause of nephrotic syndrome in children; associated with infections or vaccinations; presents with generalized anasarca, ascites, and sometimes hematuria; hypoalbuminemia (< 3 g/dL) and hypercholesterolemia; BUN and creatinine slightly elevated; UA shows proteinuria (> 3.5 g/dL) and hypercalciuria; renal biopsy is normal on light and immunofluorescence microscopy; electron microscopy reveals flattening of the foot processes of epithelial cells; treat with corticosteroids; complications include renal vein thrombosis (due to hypercoagulable state), spontaneous bacterial peritonitis, and chronic renal disease.

POSTSTREPTOCOCCAL GLOMERULONEPHRITIS

◘ Membranoproliferative Glomerulonephritis

Idiopathic diffuse glomerular disease; presents with anasarca, hematuria, and hypertension; elevated BUN and creatinine; hypocomplementemia; UA shows fatty casts and proteins; treat with aspirin; renal transplant is the only definitive therapy.

POSTSTREPTOCOCCAL GLOMERULONEPHRITIS

ID/CC	A 4-year-old boy is evaluated for **difficulty running.**
HPI	The mother states that her son was one of the last children to walk, adding that he is **unable to keep up with his friends.** He is also **unable to jump or hop normally,** and he **climbs stairs one foot at a time.** He must use his hands when standing up from the floor (= GOWERS' MANEUVER).
PE	VS: normal. PE: **positive Gowers' sign** (weakness of lower back and pelvic girdle musculature); **enlarged firm, rubbery calves** (= PSEUDOHYPERTROPHY).
Labs	**Serum CK elevated to 20–100 times normal.** EMG: myopathy. Muscle biopsy shows fibers of varying size with replacement by fat and connective tissue; **dystrophin deficiency.**
Imaging	N/A
Pathogenesis	Duchenne's muscular dystrophy (DMD), or **pseudohypertrophic muscular dystrophy,** is an **X-linked recessive disorder** caused by **mutations in the dystrophin gene, a gene that codes for a sarcolemmal protein.** DMD is characterized by **profound progressive muscle weakness** that is **first observed in the proximal muscles.** Patients are generally delayed in their walking and demonstrate significant difficulty running and jumping. At a young age, their calf muscles hypertrophy, but the hypertrophic muscle is eventually replaced by fat and connective tissue. As the children age, they require braces to walk and eventually are confined to a wheelchair. Additionally, boys suffer from chest wall deformities, further impairing their respiratory performance and placing them at risk for fatal pulmonary infections by 16–18 years of age.
Epidemiology	DMD has an incidence of approximately 3 in 10,000 and arises **almost exclusively in boys.**
Management	**Prednisone** may slow disease progression. Patients should also receive **orthotic and orthopedic treatments.** Parents should be referred for **genetic counseling.**
Complications	Intellectual impairment (mean IQ approximately 85), kyphoscoliosis, cardiomyopathy, cardiac arrhythmias,

DUCHENNE'S MUSCULAR DYSTROPHY

CHF, pulmonary infections, and respiratory failure.

Associated Diseases   N/A

···

47.   **DUCHENNE'S MUSCULAR
                            DYSTROPHY**

ID/CC	A **3-year-old child** is admitted with an **abdominal mass** that was detected on routine exam.
HPI	The child is **asymptomatic**, has no history of hematuria, has never been diagnosed as hypertensive, and does not suffer from any obvious congenital malformation. Neither parent reports any familial disease.
PE	VS: normal BP. PE: appears normal; weight and height normal for age; abdomen appears distended; large, **firm, nontender intra-abdominal mass** palpated toward the right, not crossing midline.
Labs	CBC/UA: normal. LFTs: normal. Mass biopsy reveals sheets of **small oval cells with scant cytoplasm** and primitive glomerular and tubular structures occasionally seen; urinary vanillylmandelic acid (VMA) levels normal (to rule out neuroblastoma).
Imaging	US-Abdomen: a massive **intra-abdominal tumor arising out of the right kidney.** CT-Abdomen: (used to define extent of local invasion and involvement of inferior vena cava): normal IVC.
Pathogenesis	Wilms' tumor is a neoplastic disease of unknown etiology. Karyotypic abnormalities, particularly deletions of the short arm of chromosome 11, may be etiologically important. The tumor results from **neoplastic embryonal renal cells** of the metanephros. Both Wilms' tumor and retinoblastoma are postulated to evolve through two distinct "hits" to the host genome. There is prezygotic (germ-line) inheritance of the first hit. The postzygotic (somatic) mutation, the second hit, induces malignancy in the tissue rendered susceptible by the first hit.
Epidemiology	Wilms' tumor is the **second most common abdominal neoplasm** in children (behind neuroblastoma) and occurs with equal frequency in boys and girls. The usual age of diagnosis is between four months and six years, with the **median age** being about **three years.** Ten percent of patients have bilateral Wilms' tumors. Children with sporadic aniridia, hemihypertrophy, and GU abnormalities are at increased risk for Wilms' tumor. **WAGR syndrome** is characterized by Wilms' tumor, aniridia, ambiguous genitalia, and mental retardation.

Management	Requires **surgical resection** of the primary tumor and any lymph nodes or selected metastases. **Radiotherapy** is used to treat residual local disease and selected metastatic foci. **Chemotherapy** varies in duration and intensity depending on the stage and histology, but regimens usually include **actinomycin D** and **vincristine**.
Complications	N/A
Associated Diseases	◼ **Neuroblastoma** A malignant neoplasm arising from immature cells of the adrenal medulla (neural crest cell origin) that secrete catecholamines; occurs in children < 5 years; presents with an abdominal mass; elevated urinary catecholamines; CT shows mass obliterating adrenal gland; treat by surgical resection and chemotherapy.

ID/CC	A 1-year-old **girl** is evaluated for a **limp**.
HPI	She has just begun to walk, and the parents noticed a marked **deficit in her left hip and leg.** She is **the first-born child** of a healthy couple of **Navajo Indian** origin. Directed questioning discloses that the child was born in a **breech presentation.**
PE	Asymmetry of gluteal folds (present in 40% of normal newborns); **inability to passively abduct the left flexed hip to 90 degrees;** leg in external rotation; lordosis and **waddling gait;** abduction of affected thigh causes palpable click as femoral head returns to acetabulum (= ORTOLANI'S SIGN); with hips kept in 90-degree flexion; level of knee height is lower in affected side (= GALEAZZI'S SIGN with unilateral involvement); hip falls to unaffected side when child stands on foot of affected side (= TRENDELENBURG'S SIGN).
Labs	Normal.
Imaging	**[A]** A different case with bilateral femoral head dislocation and shallow **dysplastic acetabula** (1). **[B]** XR-Pelvis: a different case with delayed appearance (1) of the femoral ossification center on the right side. (X-rays are not useful before six weeks of age. US is therefore more sensitive for diagnosis in neonates, since the ossification center is not seen on radiographs.)
Pathogenesis	An abnormal relationship between the head of the femur and the acetabular articular surface due to mechanical defects (breech presentation, first born, oligohydramnios) that produce instability leading to dislocation of the hip joint. Also called **developmental dysplasia of the hip.** Dislocation may be partial or complete.
Epidemiology	Occurs in 1 in 1,000 births, with a higher incidence found in Navajo Indians and a low incidence among blacks. Affects **females** more frequently than males and first-born children more than subsequent pregnancies. Occurs more frequently on the left side and is bilateral in one-fifth of all cases. It is associated with **breech** presentations, congenital torticollis, and spina bifida.
Management	The key to correct management of congenital dislocation of the hip lies in **early diagnosis;** the sooner it is

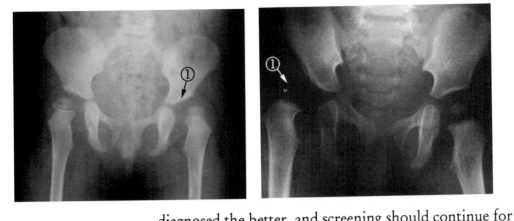

diagnosed the better, and screening should continue for at least one year following diagnosis. The newborn exam is the most important one from a diagnostic perspective, but follow-up exams are also needed to detect later-onset congenital hip dislocation. In children < 3 months of age, **a Frejka pillow, a Pavlik harness, or a spica cast** is used for three months to keep the hip flexed and abducted with the femoral head in place. Forced abduction is undesirable owing to the risk of aseptic necrosis of the femoral head. In children > 3 months, an adductor myotomy or elongation is needed for reduction, followed by a spica cast for longer periods. In children > 18 months, osteotomy and open reduction are needed. Success is inversely proportional to age at diagnosis.

Complications Flattening of the acetabular articular surface with osteoarthritis of the joint, aseptic necrosis of the femoral head, swaying (unilateral involvement) or waddling (bilateral involvement) gait, and limping.

Associated Diseases ◻ **Osteomyelitis** A pyogenic bone infection most commonly caused by *S. aureus;* presents with pain, swelling, warmth, redness, and immobility of joint; elevated ESR; MR reveals new osteoblastic periosteal bone formation (= INVOLUCRUM) with trapping of necrotic bone (= SEQUESTRUM); treat with surgical debridement and at least six weeks of IV antibiotics.

◻ **Slipped Capital Femoral Epiphysis** The most common deformity occurring in adolescence; the proximal femoral metaphysis externally rotates and displaces anteriorly from the capital femoral epiphysis; presents with an antalgic gait and severe hip or knee pain; XR shows displacement or widened epiphyseal plate; treat by fixation of the epiphysis to the metaphysis with a cannulated screw.

ID/CC	A **2-year-old girl** is brought to the pediatrician with **swelling and pain in her right knee of three months' duration.**
HPI	Yesterday she developed a **rash** and became fatigued. Her mother has also noticed "redness" of the eyes (due to uveitis).
PE	VS: normal. PE: micrognathia; slit-lamp exam shows **uveitis**; right knee swollen, erythematous, and tender to palpation with **limitation of passive and active movements.**
Labs	CBC: normocytic, normochromic anemia. **ESR elevated; ANA positive; rheumatoid factor (RF) negative** (RF may be positive in polyarticular type).
Imaging	XR-Knee: soft tissue swelling; osteopenia.
Pathogenesis	Juvenile rheumatoid arthritis (JRA) is idiopathic in nature but has an immune component. Articular involvement of **at least one joint for at least six weeks** in a child **younger than 16 years** is necessary for diagnosis. Several infectious agents, including rubella, herpesvirus, and EBV, have been implicated. JRA is divided into three types: pauciarticular, polyarticular, and systemic. The **pauciarticular form** is the most common variety and generally presents with involvement of one joint, usually the knee. The ankles are also commonly affected. It is associated with HLA-DR5 and uveitis and is more common in girls. The **polyarticular form** is associated with HLA-DR4 and involves five or more joints with symmetrical involvement; there is a female predisposition, and rheumatoid factor is usually negative. **Systemic disease** (= STILL'S DISEASE) is associated with high, spiking fever, rash, leukocytosis with neutrophilia, splenomegaly, and markedly elevated ESR. ANA and rheumatoid factor are usually negative.
Epidemiology	More common in **girls**; onset is before 16 years of age. Half a million patients are diagnosed with JRA each year in the U.S. There are two peaks of incidence: from 1 to 3 years and from 8 to 12 years.
Management	**Aspirin** for pauciarticular variety unless chickenpox or flu is suspected (risk of Reye's syndrome).

JUVENILE RHEUMATOID ARTHRITIS

Polyarticular/systemic-onset disease may require **chloroquine, methotrexate,** or other **immunosuppressive agents.** If carditis or hemolytic anemia is present, **steroids** may be used.

Complications Chronicity, recurrence, disability, chronic uveitis, and progression to ankylosing spondylitis and iridocyclitis.

Associated Diseases

◻ **Lyme Disease** Caused by the spirochete *Borrelia burgdorferi;* the vector is the *Ixodes* tick; presents with a migrating, target-shaped, erythematous rash called erythema migrans as well as with lymphadenopathy and arthritis; positive IgM ELISA for *B. burgdorferi;* treat with doxycycline.

◻ **Rheumatic Fever** Complication of group A streptococcal infection, secondary to autoantibodies directed against joints and heart valves; presents > 1 week after throat infection with migratory polyarthritis, endocarditis, and rash; antistreptococcal antibodies (e.g., ASO); treat with aspirin and penicillin; complications include permanent valvular disease.

◻ **Septic Arthritis** *S. aureus* is the most common cause; presents with red, swollen, and tender knee; leukocytosis; joint aspiration shows yellowish synovial fluid; XR of the knee shows swelling and effusion; treat with antibiotics appropriate to the organism found on joint aspiration.

ID/CC	A **7-year-old boy** is seen for a **limp in his right leg** of about three months' duration with no apparent cause.
HPI	He also complains of **groin pain** that **radiates to the inner thigh** (pain in slipped capital femoral epiphysis is referred to the medial knee). He denies any trauma or recent infections.
PE	VS: normal. PE: well developed and well nourished; **right leg shorter** than left; **tenderness and muscle spasticity** over right **hip joint**; decreased range of motion on abduction and internal rotation of affected hip.
Labs	Unremarkable.
Imaging	**[A]** XR-Hip: small femoral head epiphysis with increased density (= SCLEROSIS). Partial vs. total collapse of the femoral head can also be seen on radiographs in advanced stages of disease. **[B]** XR-Hip: another case with severe flattening and sclerosis of the right femoral head (1). MR (preferred for making diagnosis): marrow edema and fracture line in the femoral head. Nuc: abnormal uptake in the femoral head.
Pathogenesis	Idiopathic type of avascular necrosis of bone. The process is self-limited for a period of up to three years. Roughly half of all patients recover fully with bone revascularization; half will have permanent hip deformity.
Epidemiology	**More common in boys** than in girls; primarily affects children **between 3 and 12 years.**
Management	Weight bearing may be permitted with the use of a **Petrie walking cast** in which the joint is braced so that proper remodeling of bone can occur (in **abduction and medial rotation**). Moderate to severe cases are treated with **acetabular** or **femoral osteotomy.**
Complications	N/A
Associated Diseases	◘ **Congenital Hip Dislocation** An idiopathic condition likely due to joint laxity or intrauterine position; can be unilateral or bilateral; presents with inability to abduct the limb; abduction and external rotation produce characteristic clicking noise during physical exam; treat with splint devices (Pavlik harness) to assist normal

LEGG-CALVE-PERTHES DISEASE

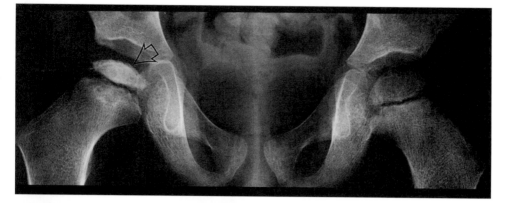

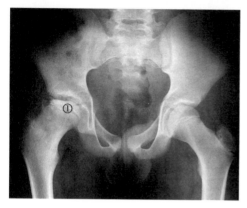

reduction of dislocation during growth; complications of untreated disease include deformed joint and limb.

◻ **Slipped Capital Femoral Epiphysis** The most common deformity occurring in adolescence; the proximal femoral metaphysis externally rotates and displaces anteriorly from the capital femoral epiphysis; presents with an antalgic gait and severe hip or knee pain; XR shows displacement or widened epiphyseal plate; treat by fixation of the epiphysis to the metaphysis with a cannulated screw.

ID/CC	A 6-year-old child is brought to the ER by his parents with acute **pain and deformity** of his left arm (due to fracture) that began during warm-up exercises for physical education class (minor trauma).
HPI	The child has sustained **four fractures** in the last **two years**.
PE	VS: normal. PE: short for age; **blue sclerae;** corneal opacities; keratoconus; partial **conduction deafness** in both ears (most common after 10 years of age); **abnormal teeth** (= DENTINOGENESIS IMPERFECTA); hand and finger joints show **increased elasticity; kyphosis and scoliosis present.** [A] Another case with multiple skeletal deformities.
Labs	Unremarkable.
Imaging	XR: generalized **osteopenia with radiolucency of long bones;** wormian bones in the skull; vertebrae appear flattened; **poorly healed old fractures;** acute **left humeral fracture;** significant bony bowing and angular deformity may be present.
Pathogenesis	Also called **brittle bone disease,** it is an **autosomal-dominant** disorder of connective tissue characterized by a mutation in the gene that codes for **type I collagen,** resulting in abnormal collagen synthesis and deficient ossification and **frequent fractures** in children. Patients frequently present with **blue sclerae and conduction deafness,** abnormal platelet function, and hyperkinetic circulation.
Epidemiology	A rare disorder. Fractures generally do not occur before the first year of life.
Management	Treatment is **supportive,** with orthopedic treatment of fractures and deformities along with physiotherapy and rehabilitation. Growth hormone and calcitonin are investigational. Ascorbic acid and calcium are usually given. Prevention through **genetic counseling** is necessary, since this is an autosomal-dominant disorder.
Complications	**Skull fracture during delivery;** multiple fractures and **recurrent joint dislocations.**
Associated Diseases	N/A

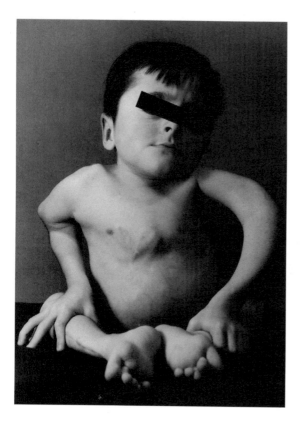

OSTEOGENESIS IMPERFECTA

ID/CC	A **1-year-old** male is brought to the emergency room with a swollen left thigh.
HPI	The mother, who appears very concerned, **states that the child fell from the bed.** She is a divorcée who is now living with a new boyfriend.
PE	Child looks **apprehensive** and begins to cry even when touched gently; **retinal hemorrhages** present; tender swelling seen over left thigh; **multiple bruises seen over body** in various stages of resolution (mother suspects a clotting defect).
Labs	Coagulation profile normal.
Imaging	XR-Left Thigh: spiral fracture of the femur. Skeletal Survey: **old fractures** in the humerus, both tibia, and ribs, seen in **different stages of healing** (highly suggestive of child abuse). Bone density normal (metabolically normal bones).
Pathogenesis	**Injuries intentionally perpetrated by a caretaker that result in morbidity or mortality constitute physical abuse.** Failure to provide a child with appropriate food, clothing, medical care, schooling, and a safe environment constitutes neglect. Instances that should arouse suspicion of abuse include cuts and bruises in low-trauma areas such as the buttocks or back, fractures that occur before ambulation, multiple fractures in different stages of healing in metabolically normal bones (thereby excluding osteogenesis imperfecta), **multiple bruises over the body in the absence of any bleeding disorder,** injury that is inconsistent with the stated history or delay in obtaining appropriate medical care, spiral fractures in young children, and **retinal hemorrhages** that result from vigorous shaking ("shaken baby syndrome").
Epidemiology	Almost half of the children who receive medical attention as a result of physical abuse are < 1 year, and the vast majority are preschoolers. Parents, mothers' boyfriends, and stepparents are the most frequent perpetrators. Mortality is 5%.
Management	Health care workers are **required by law to report any suspicion** of child abuse or neglect to state protection agencies. Physicians are not liable for any damages even

CHILD ABUSE (PHYSICAL)

if the abuse is disproved later. Suitable orthopedic treatment for injuries.

Complications	N/A
Associated Diseases	□ **Hemophilia** An X-linked genetic defect of factor VIII (= HEMOPHILIA A) or of factor IX (= HEMOPHILIA B); presents in young children with hemorrhage, hemarthroses, and ecchymoses secondary to minor trauma; prolonged PTT and low factor VIII levels; treat with recombinant factor VIII or IX, transfusions as needed; complications include massive hemorrhage or acquisition of infections (e.g., HIV, hepatitis viruses) via blood and blood products.

□ **von Willebrand's Disease** An inherited (mostly autosomal-dominant) disorder caused by a deficiency of von Willebrand factor (vWF); presents with episodic mucosal, GI, and dental bleeding and easy bruisability; increased bleeding time, prolonged PTT, and decreased ristocetin cofactor and factor VIII antigen; treat with avoidance of aspirin, use of desmopressin acetate, factor VIII concentrates that contain functional vWF and cryoprecipitate. |

ID/CC	A 10-year-old male presents with chest congestion, **cough, difficulty breathing, and wheezing.**
HPI	His symptoms started four days ago when he caught a **cold.** He is **allergic to cats and pollen** and had **eczema** during infancy as well as **allergic rhinitis.** He has had repeated attacks of wheezing over the years (asthma), one of which required hospitalization. His **mother and maternal uncle** suffer from severe **asthma.**
PE	VS: slight fever; **tachypnea;** tachycardia. PE: **dyspnea** with increased respiratory effort; **nasal mucosa** boggy and **pale** (due to allergy); uses **accessory muscles of respiration; expiratory wheezes and high-pitched sibilant rhonchi** heard throughout lung fields; **prolongation of expiration; hyperresonance** to percussion.
Labs	CBC: leukocytosis with lymphocytosis (viral infection) and **eosinophilia** (allergic component). Increased serum IgE. ABGs: **respiratory alkalosis, hypocarbia, and hypoxemia** (in severe cases, CO_2 retention [respiratory acidosis]). PFTs: increased total lung capacity and residual volume; **decreased FEV_1/FVC** (reversible with beta-agonists).
Imaging	CXR: lung **hyperinflation** with flattened diaphragm; peribronchial cuffing and linear atelectasis in both bases.
Pathogenesis	Asthma is characterized by **episodic airway hyperreactivity** and inflammation. It may be intrinsic or initiated by an **allergen** (type I hypersensitivity reaction). One observes reversible constriction of airway smooth muscle, hypersecretion of mucus, edema, inflammatory cell (particularly mast cell) infiltration, and epithelial desquamation. In atopic asthma, a **biphasic response** is frequently observed. An acute phase is marked by immediate hypersensitivity and mast cell degranulation, with return toward baseline within one hour. Recurrences, which are characterized by more severe airway obstruction, arise 3–8 hours after initial exposure.
Epidemiology	Affects 5% of U.S. population. May be **extrinsic** (allergic; best prognosis) or **intrinsic** (idiosyncratic; no hypersensitivity). Fifty percent of patients outgrow asthma after puberty. **Associated with** hay fever,

ATOPIC ASTHMA

rhinitis, urticaria, aspirin sensitivity (nasal polyps), eczema, and family history.

Management   Acute management includes **oxygen, bronchodilators** (beta-agonists or anticholinergics), and **corticosteroids;** subcutaneous adrenaline in severe instances. Chronic management involves avoidance of allergens, regularly inhaled bronchodilators or steroids, systemic steroids, cromolyn, or theophylline (check blood levels). Start **anti-inflammatory agents (cromolyn, steroids)** if the patient is symptomatic > 2 times a week or has nocturnal symptoms > 2 times a month. Leukotriene antagonists can be used as adjuncts.

Complications   Pneumothorax, pulsus paradoxus (very severe asthma), orthopnea, and respiratory failure.

Associated Diseases

☐ **Bronchiolitis** Most commonly caused by RSV in infants; presents with wheezing, nasal flaring, rhonchi, and congestion; lymphocytosis and hypoxemia; positive culture of throat swab; CXR shows hyperinflation and atelectasis; treat with humidified oxygen and fluid management, ribavirin for children with underlying heart or lung disease.

☐ **Churg–Strauss Angiitis** Idiopathic systemic small- and medium-vessel granulomatous vasculitis; presents with asthma and hypertension; eosinophilia, elevated BUN and creatinine, and proteinuria; CXR shows bilateral infiltrates; treat with corticosteroids.

☐ **Atopy** Idiopathic propensity to IgE-mediated allergic reactions, seen in asthmatics and patients with dermatitis, with strong familial inheritance; presents with rhinitis, asthma, and eczema; treatment is avoidance of allergic triggers, supportive use of antihistamines, bronchodilators, and topical corticosteroids.

☐ **Atopic Dermatitis** An idiopathic, chronic, IgE-mediated skin inflammation; presents with intense pruritus, lichenification secondary to scratching, erythema, and scaling; treat with topical corticosteroids, hydrating creams, and removal of potential allergens; complications include secondary infection.

ID/CC	A 4-year-old **white** male is brought to the pediatrician with complaints of **frequent, fatty, foul-smelling, bulky stools** (malabsorption) of about three months' duration, coupled with a **productive cough** (greenish, foul-smelling sputum), high fever, and difficulty breathing for the past day.
HPI	He has a history suggestive of **meconium ileus** and rectal prolapse as well as **recurrent pulmonary infections** (inspissated mucus cannot be cleared from respiratory tract). He has also shown **failure to thrive** despite substantial caloric intake (due to malabsorption). A sibling has similar symptoms.
PE	VS: fever (38.4 C); tachycardia; **tachypnea.** PE: **pale** and undernourished; **low weight and height for age;** nasal exam reveals **polyps** on left side (20% of cases); barrel-shaped chest; **dullness to percussion** in right lower lung field (due to pneumonia); crepitant rales with crackles and rhonchi; hepatomegaly.
Labs	CBC: **anemia** (Hb 8.3) with micro- and macrocytosis (folate and iron deficiency due to malabsorption); **leukocytosis** with neutrophilia. Hyperglycemia (pancreatic endocrine insufficiency); hypoalbuminemia; **elevated sweat chloride** levels; **sputum culture yields** *Pseudomonas.* PFTs: increased residual volume and total lung capacity. ABGs: hypoxemia.
Imaging	**[A]** CXR: an older patient shows hyperinflation; ring shadows (suggesting bronchiectasis). **[B]** CT-Chest: another patient with thick-walled, dilated bronchi in the left lower lobe from recurrent pneumonia.
Pathogenesis	An **autosomal-recessive** disorder affecting the exocrine glands; due to a mutation of chromosome 7q carrying the **cystic fibrosis transmembrane conductance regulator (CFTR)** gene. The mutation produces alterations in chloride and water transport in epithelial cells, with secretion of abnormal mucus (thick and viscous) that plugs gland ducts (mostly in the pancreas and bronchi), leading to chronic pancreatitis and bronchiectasis. CF is characterized by recurrent URIs, lower respiratory tract infections (commonly with *Pseudomonas* and *S. aureus*), lung scarring, and

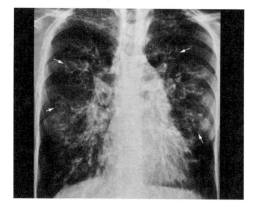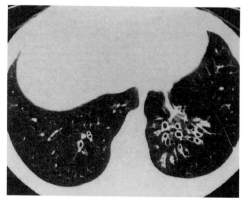

pneumothorax.

Epidemiology A common genetic disease in Caucasians. CF is the principal cause of COPD in children, with an incidence of **1 in 2,500 whites;** 1 in 25 is a carrier of a mutation in the CFTR gene. **Median survival** is 29 years.

Management General management includes a **low-fat diet,** vitamins, minerals (salt), and enzyme supplements. Steroid use is controversial; **recombinant human DNase** renders mucus less viscous (side effect is hoarseness). In the presence of **pseudomonal pneumonia,** give ticarcillin/clavulanate, ceftazidime, or piperacillin. **Lung transplantation** is an option but is costly and associated with a high rate of bronchiolitis obliterans. Prevention of lung infections includes **immunizations against** *Pneumococcus* **and influenza, chest physiotherapy,** postural drainage, antibiotics, and bronchodilators.

Complications Increased risk of GI tract malignancy, biliary cirrhosis, **pancreatic exocrine insufficiency,** gallstones, pulmonary fibrosis, exudative retinopathy, optic neuritis, diabetes, bleeding/coagulation problems, night blindness, and osteomalacia; in neonates, heat shock, rectal prolapse, and **meconium ileus** occur.

Associated Diseases ▣ **Bronchiectasis** Dilatation of bronchioles secondary to chronic inflammation; most commonly seen in chronic infection (e.g., tuberculosis, fungal) or cystic fibrosis; presents with chronic productive cough, repeated pneumonias, hemoptysis, and crackles on exam; CXR reveals "honeycombing" and "tram tracking" due to bronchial wall thickening; treat with aggressive chest physiotherapy, antibiotics for acute and chronic

infection, home oxygen; complications include lung and
metastatic abscesses and amyloidosis.

ID/CC	A 14-year-old girl is found lying semiconscious in her room by her mother.
HPI	The mother found a suicide note and an empty **pesticide** bottle lying in the room. The girl **vomited and passed loose stools** several times while being brought to the hospital.
PE	VS: **bradycardia** (HR 50). PE: drowsy and dehydrated; breath smells strongly of a **pesticide; pupils are pinpoint** with **hypersalivation; lacrimation.**
Labs	Red cell cholinesterase activity level < 25% of normal.
Imaging	N/A
Pathogenesis	Organophosphates and carbamates are widely used as pesticides. They **inhibit the enzyme acetylcholinesterase,** decreasing the breakdown of acetylcholine at cholinergic synapses. Whereas the organophosphates may cause permanent inhibition of the enzyme, carbamates have a transient and reversible effect. Many of these agents are well **absorbed through intact skin.**
Epidemiology	Individuals may be exposed accidentally while working with or transporting the chemicals or as a result of accidental or intentional ingestion.
Management	As an initial step in management, it is important to immediately remove all contaminated clothing and wash all exposed areas with **soap and water.** Specific therapy includes administration of **atropine and pralidoxime (2-PAM).** Atropine is not a pharmacologic antidote but can reverse excessive muscarinic stimulation, thereby **alleviating bradycardia, abdominal cramps, bronchospasm, and hypersalivation** (it does not reverse muscle weakness). All patients should also be given pralidoxime, since it restores the enzyme acetylcholinesterase. In those who go untreated, the organophosphates binding to acetylcholinesterase may become irreversible (the so-called aging effect). Because carbamates have a transient effect, pralidoxime therapy is not needed.
Complications	N/A

ORGANOPHOSPHATE AND CARBAMATE POISONING

Associated Diseases

□ **Reye's Syndrome** An idiopathic disorder linked to children with influenza B and varicella infection who have been treated with salicylates; presents with coma, fever, and hepatomegaly; impaired liver function; CT shows cerebral edema; treat with emergent liver transplantation.

ORGANOPHOSPHATE AND CARBAMATE POISONING

From the authors of *Underground Clinical Vignettes*

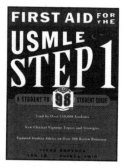

A true classic used by over 200,000 students around the world. The '99 edition features details on the new computerized test, new color plates and thoroughly updated high-yield facts and book reviews. Bi-directional links with the *Underground Clinical Vignettes Step 1* series. ISBN 0-8385-2612-8.

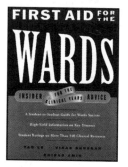

This high-yield student-to-student guide is designed to help students make the transition from the basic sciences to the hospital wards and succeed on their clinical rotations. The book features an orientation to the hospital environment, tips on being an effective and efficient junior medical student, student-proven advice tailored to each core rotation, a database of high-yield clinical facts, and recommendations for clinical pocket books, texts, and references.
ISBN 0-8385-2595-4.

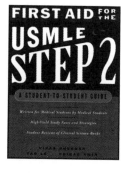

This entirely rewritten second edition now follows in the footsteps of *First Aid for the USMLE Step 1*. Features an exam preparation guide geared to the new computerized test, basic science and clinical high-yield facts, color plates and ratings of USMLE Step 2 books and software. Bi-directional links with the *Underground Clinical Vignettes Step 2* series.

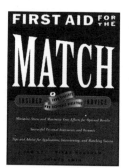

This top rated (5 stars, *Doody Review*) student-to-student guide helps medical students effectively and efficiently navigate the residency application process, helping them make the most of their limited time, money, and energy. The book draws on the advice and experiences of successful student applicants as well as residency directors. Also featured are application and interview tips tailored to each specialty, successful personal statements and CVs with analyses, current trends, and common interview questions with suggested strategies for responding. ISBN 0-8385-2596-2.

The *First Aid* series by Appleton & Lange...the review book leader.
Available through your local health sciences bookstore !